Tangled Minds

Understanding Alzheimer's Disease and Other Dementias

MURIEL R. GILLICK, M.D.

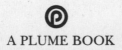

ⓟ

A PLUME BOOK

A NOTE TO THE READER

The ideas, procedures, and suggestions contained in this book are not intended as a substitute for medical treatment by a physician. The reader should regularly consult a physician in matters related to health.

PLUME
Published by the Penguin Group
Penguin Putnam Inc., 375 Hudson Street, New York, New York 10014, U.S.A.
Penguin Books Ltd, 27 Wrights Lane, London W8 5TZ, England
Penguin Books Australia Ltd, Ringwood, Victoria, Australia
Penguin Books Canada Ltd, 10 Alcorn Avenue, Toronto, Ontario,
  Canada M4V 3B2
Penguin Books (N.Z.) Ltd, 182–190 Wairau Road, Auckland 10,
  New Zealand

Penguin Books Ltd, Registered Offices: Harmondsworth,
  Middlesex, England

Published by Plume, a member of Penguin Putnam Inc.
Previously published in a Dutton edition.

First Plume Printing, April, 1999
10 9 8 7 6 5 4 3 2 1

Ⓟ REGISTERED TRADEMARK—MARCA REGISTRADA

The Library of Congress has catalogued the Dutton edition as follows:
Gillick, Muriel R.
    Tangled minds : understanding Alzheimer's disease and other
dementias / Muriel R. Gillick.
        p.   cm.
    Includes bibliographical references
    ISBN 0-525-94145-2
          0-452-27647-0 (pbk.)
    1. Alzheimer's disease—Popular works.   2. Presenile dementia—
Popular works.   3. Health education.   I. Title.
    RC523.2.G55   1998
    616.8'31—dc21   97-34928
                                                                 CIP

Printed in the United States of America
Original hardcover design by Leonard Telesca

BOOKS ARE AVAILABLE AT QUANTITY DISCOUNTS WHEN USED TO PROMOTE PRODUCTS OR SERVICES. FOR INFORMATION PLEASE WRITE TO PREMIUM MARKETING DIVISION, PENGUIN PUTNAM INC., 375 HUDSON STREET, NEW YORK, NEW YORK 10014.

As our elderly population grows dramatically, more and more families are faced with an aging parent or spouse who suffers from dementia, a disease that afflicts more than four million Americans. In *Tangled Minds*, Dr. Muriel R. Gillick, a Harvard Medical School professor and specialist on aging, gives us a comprehensive guide to coping with Alzheimer's disease and other dementias, from diagnosis to treatment and beyond. With insight and compassion, she provides the latest information on:

• Understanding the wide range of disorders that lead to a progressive loss of memory, language skills, and the capacity to solve the most basic problems of daily life

• Revolutionary discoveries and medications

• Housing alternatives

• Costs of specialized care

• And more

MURIEL R. GILLICK, M.D., is a physician specializing in the care of the elderly and medical ethics. She is assistant professor of medicine and director of the Geriatrics Program at Harvard Medical School, as well as staff physician at the Hebrew Rehabilitation Center for the Aged and at the Beth Israel Deaconess Medical Center in Boston. Winner of the Will Solimene Award for excellence in medical communications, she lives outside Boston with her husband and three sons.

To Daniel, Jeremy, and Jonathan,
in the hope they will be spared.

Contents

Acknowledgments

There is no Sylvia Truman, but I am indebted to the many patients who have gone into creating both Sylvia and the other characters in this book who have dementia. I also am grateful to the families of my Alzheimer's patients for teaching me so much—about the pain and the occasional joys of caregiving, about hope and denial, and about what dementia is really like.

Thanks to Robert Butler, John Growdon, and Robert Katzman for granting me interviews. Thanks also to my colleagues who read part or all of the manuscript and repeatedly rescued me from errors and misstatements: Katherine Hesse, Martha Holstein, Ruth Kandel, Susan Mitchell, and Ann Sheehan.

The Hebrew Rehabilitation Center for Aged, where I worked throughout the gestation of this book, graciously gave me the flexibility necessary to write while simultaneously providing me with an ample supply of patients with dementia to help populate my stories.

My agent, Jill Grinberg, not only supported the project from the outset but also remained interested and helpful throughout the process. My editor at Dutton, Deb Brody, supplied me just enough positive feedback along the way to sustain me; her incisive comments have made this a better book.

Finally, I would not have written this book without the encouragement of my husband, Larry. He knows that I am happiest when I write about my work, and he is forever urging me to turn the stories I bring home to him into another book.

Introduction

When actress Rita Hayworth was diagnosed with Alzheimer's disease, her daughter, Princess Yasmin Aga Khan, wrote an appeal to then president Ronald Reagan. She wrote about the devastating nature of the disease, and urged him to devote more federal funds to its eradication. Reagan answered her letter in May 1983:

"Dear Princess Yasmin. Like most Americans, my true understanding of the tragedy called Alzheimer's disease is relatively recent. For too long this insidious, indiscriminate killer of mind and life has gone undetected while the families of its victims have gone unaided."[1]

Reagan announced that government funding for research on Alzheimer's would be increased from $17 million to $25 million for the 1984 fiscal year. Twelve years later, in an open letter to the American public, Ronald Reagan revealed that he had Alzheimer's disease.

Once known as "the great communicator," Reagan retained his way with words even as dementia attacked his memory and reasoning capacity: "I now begin the journey that will lead me into the sunset of my life," he wrote by hand, in his widely reprinted letter. "I know that for America there will always be a bright dawn ahead." More to the point, he stated: "I have recently been told that I am one of the millions of Americans . . . afflicted with Alzheimer's disease." He continued: "In opening our hearts, we hope this might promote greater awareness of this condition. . . . Unfortunately as Alzheimer's progresses, the family often bears a heavy burden. I only wish that there was some way I could spare Nancy from this painful experience."[2]

Five months later, the news media reported a conversation between Nancy Reagan and a friend, in which she commented that her husband had seen the White House on television but did not recall having lived there. Seven months later, the Reagans attended a dinner at a celebrity restaurant in Los Angeles. As the former president left, the other diners began applauding, as was their custom. On that evening, Reagan could not understand why they were clapping. He did not remember having been president.[3]

Exactly a year after the public announcement of Reagan's diagnosis, a new Alzheimer's disease research institute was created in Reagan's name. Its mission is "to accelerate the discovery and development of treatments and preventions for Alzheimer's disease by increasing information exchange, technology transfer and alliance among investigators." Billing itself as the largest private sponsor of research on Alzheimer's, the Reagan Research Institute was established under the aegis of the country's major voluntary, lay advocacy organization dedicated to all facets of Alzheimer's disease. Its first coup was to recruit to the position of director Dr. Zaven Khachaturian, who had headed the neurosciences section of the National Institute on Aging virtually since its inception in 1975.[4]

During the same twelve-month span, researchers in the Alzheimer field declared they had found the Holy Grail they had been pursuing for ten years. The elusive goal was the gene responsible for a rare form of Alzheimer's disease—a purely genetic variant that afflicts only one hundred extended families worldwide. The gene's discovery (together with the identification of the gene for another variant within a few months) meant that virtually all types of genetic Alzheimer's disease had been pinned down, the flawed DNA literally spelled out. The confidence of the scientists who made the discoveries was unbounded: "Once we get this gene . . . we are going to understand the bulk of the Alzheimer's disease process . . . because here is a gene that leads to the earliest onset of the disease."[5]

The Reagan saga, together with the other developments during that year between the announcement of the diagnosis and the creation of the institute bearing Reagan's name, contains all the themes of the Alzheimer story: personal loss as brain failure sets in, devastated families struggling to deal with behavioral and cognitive changes they never bargained for, scientific breakthroughs, an influential lay advocacy group, and, of course, politics.

Dementia has been called the disease of the century, the worst of all diseases.[6] It is a collection of disorders producing progressive cognitive loss in multiple domains, including memory, language, and the capacity to solve the problems of daily life. Dementia affects four million Americans: 5 percent of those over sixty-five, but nearly 50 percent of those over eighty-five. The most common type is Alzheimer's disease, accounting for 60 to 70 percent of all cases. This translates into 2.5 million cases in the United States, and over 22 million cases worldwide.[7] Because it is so common, dementia will touch the lives of us all. Even if we ourselves escape, our spouses or our friends or our parents will be afflicted.

There is yet another reason for believing that we should all come to understand what dementia is about. Beyond its effect on the victim, in addition to its effect on caregivers, and besides the costs of caring for people with dementia, a deep understanding of dementia is essential because our views toward old people in general are inextricably intertwined with our attitudes toward dementia. The demographic reality—the changing age structure of the American population, with a dramatic rise in the percentage over age sixty-five and an even more staggering rise in the percentage over age eighty— clearly has political, economic, and social consequences. As a society, we need to figure out what to do with our old people: where they should live, what kind of medical care they should receive, how to help them find meaning in their lives.

More and more voices are clamoring that we are spending too much on the elderly. Some of the protestors are realists, arguing that there is no *need* to set the retirement age at sixty-five when many older people are both eager and able to continue working considerably longer. Some of the critiques are concerned about intergenerational equity, claiming that there is not enough to go around and that children, rather than octogenarians, should be the beneficiaries of government largesse. Still others argue that there is more to life than health care—we should work toward enabling old people to lead lives they find *meaningful*, rather than just maximizing sheer survival.[8] But if changes in the Social Security system and in Medicare are inevitable—and most analysts believe the current entitlement programs are unsustainable—then surely it behooves all of us to look more closely at what aging is all about.[9]

The prevailing tendency of economists is to regard "the elderly" as a homogeneous group, except insofar as some have savings and some do not, and some are the "young old" (who are generally healthy) while increasing numbers make up the "old old" (those over eighty, who are often not so healthy). In fact, old people are heterogeneous: some are robust (afflicted perhaps by numerous ills, none of which seriously interferes with their daily functioning); some are frail (the particular medical problems they have result in their depending on assistance in such basic activities as eating, walking, or bathing); some are dying (with a diagnosis or combination of diagnoses that statistically make them almost certain to be dead within six months); and some are demented (cognitively frail). To make the kinds of decisions about how to provide care to the elderly that politicians, physicians, and the citizenry as a whole will be called on to make over the coming decades, understanding the aging condition, in all its variety, is imperative.[10]

Of all the predicaments of aging, dementia is the most frightening, the least well understood, and the most widespread. Death and dying received tremendous publicity, starting with Elisabeth Kübler-Ross's book *On Death and Dying* twenty years ago.[11] The raging controversy over physician-assisted suicide, epitomized by the fascination with Dr. Jack Kevorkian and his suicide machine, attests to the enduring concern with life's final stage. Sherwin Nuland's popular book, *How We Die*, together with extensive media attention to dying, provide the public with ample information about this phase of aging.[12] At the other end of the spectrum, vigorous old age is the norm according to retirement magazines such as *Modern Maturity* (the bimonthly put out by the American Association of Retired Persons, which boasts a membership of 33 million). Increasingly, the concept of "successful aging" permeates both professional and popular literature on the elderly—not only do some octogenarians and even centenarians remain robust, but the secret of their success is thought to be replicable in others. The physically frail elderly, like the cognitively frail or demented, are less familiar to most people. But thanks to the Americans with Disabilities Act and the climate that allowed for its passage, physical limitations of all sorts are increasingly better tolerated. Attitudes often lag behind legislation, and people with difficulty seeing or hearing or walking are still the objects of fear or scorn, but not nearly to the extent they once were. Dementia, however, remains as mysterious and horrific as ever. Despite the formidable educational efforts of the Alzheimer Association and despite the comprehensive media coverage of the Reagan diagnosis, dementia is still hidden from view. The most severely impaired individuals are sequestered in nursing homes, out of sight.

This book was born out of the belief that dementia continues to be poorly understood and from the conviction that an understanding of dementia is crucial to our coming to terms with aging. Aging is such an important part of life, and dementia such a critical variable in the aging equation, that all Americans need to learn about the realities of growing old—with and without dementia. This book is for family members of persons with dementia to learn about all facets of Alzheimer's disease. It is also for historians or sociologists of science, who will find Alzheimer's a rich case study that reveals much about how politics and culture affect science, and how science shapes our views of disease.[13] This book is for those older people who have all their faculties but worry about what the future has in store. Finally, this book is for the baby-boomer generation—those who face old age in their parents and, in the not too distant future, in themselves.

To begin to understand Alzheimer's disease, we have to start with the *experience* of the illness. Only by feeling what it is like to have the disease, at various points along its trajectory, and what it is like to live with an affected individual, can we begin to unravel the effect of our perception of dementia on our attitudes toward aging. That, of course, is my bias as a physician who takes care of older patients, many of whom have some degree of dementia. The backbone of this book is therefore the story of a single person with Alzheimer's disease over the course of her disease. There can be no surprise ending to such a story—the outcome is invariably death. But along the way, there are many twists and turns, many dilemmas, many decisions to be made. Some of the issues are concrete—where to live, what medications to take, how to make the diagnosis; others are more philosophical—how to preserve autonomy, promote dignity, and maximize quality of life.

Because the experiences of any one person with a disease are unique, my protagonist, Sylvia Truman, is a composite. She is based on a core person, embellished with features of many other people with the disease. Moreover, I have given Sylvia Truman friends and roommates who embody other characteristics of dementing illness. While I have felt free to embroider on reality, all the other people I describe are also based on a core person in my clinical practice of geriatric medicine.

The backdrop to the saga of dementia as illuminated by the story of one human being is the politics, the history, and the science of Alzheimer's disease. I have inserted a few factual asides and brief ethical discussions into Sylvia Truman's story, but every so often I step back to explore in greater depth factors that I view as crucial to an understanding of the disease. The influence of cultural attitudes toward aging on science (and vice versa) are brought into sharp relief by examining other historical periods. The effect of lay advocacy organizations and of government funding programs on the avenues pursued by Alzheimer's researchers deserves a chapter of its own. And the actual scientific developments— intertwined as they are with politics and culture—have been so remarkable and numerous as to merit another detour. After moving back and forth from Sylvia's story to the external factors that give meaning and direction to that tale, I discuss explicitly contemporary American attitudes toward aging in general and dementia in particular. In conclusion, I try to integrate the many strands of the Alzheimer story to reflect on how Alzheimer's disease *should* be viewed if American society is to arrive at a compassionate but realistic understanding of aging.

CHAPTER 1

Sunset

Sitting quietly in my waiting room were four members of the Truman family. The oldest of them was evidently my new patient, Sylvia Truman. She was wearing a tweed suit and was immaculately coifed. Her nails had been manicured and painted. She had on comfortable-appearing pumps—but definitely not old-lady shoes. Her hands were folded primly in her lap, and she was staring at the walls. Next to her was the one man in the room, her son, John Truman, I assumed, who had scheduled the appointment. He was wearing a tastefully tailored dark suit brightened by a gold and maroon tie. His attention was focused on his mother.

Opposite my patient and her son were two middle-aged women, one a shade thinner than svelte, the other veering toward the corpulent. The plumper one had the same solid build and curly hair as Mr. Truman and was undoubtedly his sister, Marcia, who had indicated on the phone she would be coming along. The thin one, whom I took to be my patient's daughter-in-law, had a magazine in her lap, which she was flipping though distractedly.

"Hello, I'm Dr. Gillick," I said as I took them all in. "I'll be with you as soon as the other members of the team arrive." All four turned toward me—first the nervous daughter-in-law, then my patient's children, and then, ever so slowly, Mrs. Truman herself, whom they had brought in for a geriatric consultation.

I was the geriatrician member of a team that also included

a social worker, nurse practitioner, and a psychiatrist. Together, we probed the mind and prodded the body of each frail older person who was scheduled for our scrutiny. To gain the maximum possible information in this three-hour evaluation, to be able to explore the social and psychological dimensions of our subject's existence, and to flesh out the portrait with an understanding of his physical environment, we asked that patients be accompanied by their significant others. Typically, this meant a spouse or children; sometimes a housekeeper or personal attendant came as well; occasionally we were graced with visits from a devoted ex-son-in-law or a neighbor or a lifelong friend.

Each consultation was carefully choreographed, and the visit by Sylvia Truman and her family was no exception. When my colleagues arrived, we introduced ourselves and laid out the plans for the afternoon. I shook Mrs. Truman's hand. She looked around anxiously, unsure what she was doing in my office. I smiled at her reassuringly and nodded in the direction of the three other adults who had followed her in. "This must be your family." She smiled back, obviously proud of her children and comforted by their presence.

John Truman introduced himself. "I'm the lawyer in the family—but I do real estate law, not malpractice." He laughed at his own joke. He managed to speak both warmly and commandingly and quickly took over as family spokesman, introducing his wife, Cynthia, and his sister, Marcia. Cynthia looked almost as anxious as the patient. A fashionable suit clothing her gaunt figure, she tapped her fingers on the seat of her chair and shifted her weight every few minutes. Marcia shared her brother's dimples and his ready smile, but her concern about her mother was more transparent than his. I would soon learn that John was every bit as distressed as his sister by his mother's growing forgetfulness, her inappropriate remarks when company was present, and a sudden indifference to personal hygiene belied by her external appearance.

I had positioned Sylvia Truman so that she was catty-corner to me. I sat behind my desk, which allowed me to take notes during the meeting. The Truman family formed an arc spanning the room, starting with Mrs. Truman and ending at the door. I turned my attention to the woman who was obviously the matriarch of her clan. "You have quite a few people concerned about you. What kinds of troubles have you had that they are worried about?" She responded as I hoped she would: there was a hint of a smile in the corners of her eyes as she warmed to being the center of attention. But the flurry of wrinkles rapidly receded as she realized that she had no idea why they were all gathered in my office.

I tried once more. "Are you having any medical problems right now?" She shook her head. "That's good! I'm glad you're feeling well. Is it all right if I ask your family what's on their minds?" She nodded, relieved to have the spotlight shifted to her children. I swiveled my chair slightly to face her son, John. He also seemed relieved, worried perhaps that I would waste precious minutes probing his mother for information. I felt I had already learned a fair amount. I suspected, though I could not yet be certain, that Sylvia Truman's problem was precisely that she did not know she had any problems.

Families came for a geriatric consultation for assorted reasons, not just for memory problems. I saw patients who suffered from recurrent falls, and patients who were humiliated by incontinence. I had patients brought in for consultation because they were sleepy all the time or because they were taking, in their view, too many medications—often the sleepy patients were sleepy *because* they were on excessive or inappropriate medications. Patients were scheduled for a consultation because of their behavior: they were apathetic or they were up all night or they were irritable and argumentative. Some came because their primary care physicians did not seem interested in issues such as personality changes or failure to get to the bathroom in time. In fact, patients in many cases had not dared to bring up their real problems with their regular physicians. Others came despite perfectly adequate medical care because they or their families were impressed by specialists and felt that a geriatrician would be a suitable addition to their already extensive collection of doctors that included a cardiologist, an orthopedist, a gynecologist, and an ophthalmologist.

The majority of the geriatric consultations centered around memory difficulties: "Mom is driving me crazy: she asks the same questions five times in five minutes" or "She's constantly losing things and accusing us of taking them from her" or

"He forgot his grandchildren's names—his doctor says it's normal for his age, but he also made three contributions to the same charity in a single week, and I'm afraid he's going to give all his money away and have to go on Medicaid." Sylvia Truman, I guessed, judging by that lost expression on her face and her inability to answer my questions, was having trouble with her memory.

"Mom's having some trouble with her memory," her son began. His mother glared at him, either disputing his claim or indicating that if it was true, he certainly should not be talking about it to me, whoever I was. He patted her hand affectionately. "It's okay, Mom, I forget things too."

"We'll sign you up for an appointment next," I chimed in. "But today it's your turn, Mrs. Truman. I just want to learn a little about you, check a few things, and see if there's anything I can do to help." I turned to John for the history, and Mrs. Truman began to relax, gradually tuning out our conversation.

The next twenty minutes were devoted to gathering information about Sylvia Truman's past medical history and about the development of her memory difficulty. It turned out that she had been a very healthy woman—she had picked up a few scars here and there, from an appendectomy as a teenager and a gallbladder removal a few years ago—and she was taking only one medication, a single pill once a day (if she remembered to take it) for high blood pressure. The social worker would obtain the details of her social circumstances; for the moment it sufficed for me to know that Sylvia Truman lived alone in a single-family house, the same house where she had raised John and Marcia, where she lived with her husband until his death from a heart attack two years ago.

It was after Mr. Truman's death that the children had begun to notice that Mom was forgetful. Most likely he had compensated for her deficits, serving as her address book and appointment calendar. He had probably covered up for her, too, cleverly devising excuses when she forgot an important family birthday or did not recognize an old friend or said something that made little sense. I saw this kind of dependency often—one spouse relying on the other to shore up a failing memory and keep up appearances. Sometimes one member of an aging couple developed physical problems and the other cognitive problems, and they complemented each other nicely. Family and friends, unless they lived with the person with the memory problems or saw her regularly, were often unaware of the change. If the mentally intact partner was hospitalized or died, the cracks in the remaining spouse began to show.

John started to describe what had happened when his father had died: how his mother could not seem to remember that her husband had died, which the family chalked up to denial; how she had forgotten to bring underwear or pajamas in her overnight bag when she went to stay with John and Cynthia at their country cottage, which they blamed on her being depressed; how her granddaughter found her circling around the one-story bungalow looking for the staircase to the bedroom, which they attributed to her being in an unfamiliar place. John's wife and sister added their own anecdotes. They had taken Mrs. Truman to her regular doctor, who prescribed an antidepressant. After that Mrs. Truman had seemed even more confused. She began calling her family in the middle of the night, convinced it was daytime. She slept in the afternoon and had trouble going to sleep at night. Her internist prescribed a sleeping pill. The confusion became a little worse.

The final straw had been when Mrs. Truman went shopping and locked herself out. She had forgotten her key and had absolutely no idea how to get inside. She concluded that she was at the wrong house and began walking, shopping bag in hand, up and down the streets, looking for her house. Two hours later, a neighbor recognized her, brought her home, and ended up calling the police when she discovered Mrs. Truman did not have her key.

I was certain now that something was very wrong with Sylvia Truman. I thought it was most likely dementia, given the gradual onset of forgetfulness and problems in both orientation and in judgment. But I would try to keep an open mind: all her symptoms could be manifestations of depression. They might be due, at least in part, to the medication she was on for her blood pressure, or to residual adverse effects from the antidepressant and the sleeping pill that were only now being cleared from her system. I moved on to the next part of the evaluation, the physical examination, while my social work colleague, Nancy Kingsley, met with the family privately to discuss other concerns they might not have voiced with Mrs. Truman present and to learn more about the family dynamics and the kind of help relatives provided.

Nancy learned that Sylvia Truman was of Italian background. Her parents had been immigrants: they had deliberately chosen a very American name for their only child to emphasize that they might be from the Old Country, but their daughter was 100 percent American. Perhaps in keeping with her family's aspirations for her, Sylvia had married a man "whose family came over on the *Mayflower*," John Truman explained. He had been the manager of a clothing store; she, just out of high school, had been a salesgirl. They courted for six months, but after the first date, according to family legend, Sylvia had made up her mind to get married. They were together for sixty-two years, through sickness and health, poverty and wealth. Mr. Truman did not approve of married women working—he believed that any self-respecting man should be able to support his family. So from their wedding day, Sylvia Truman had been a housewife and, a year later, a mother.

She had been a strict but affectionate mother. Barred from using her considerable managerial talents outside the home, she devoted her skills to domestic management. They had lost everything during the Depression—her husband's store had gone out of business and he had been unemployed—but managed to survive on odd jobs and parental largesse. When, ten years later, they regained lost ground and even saved enough for a down payment on a house, Sylvia was overjoyed. Her greatest ambition was fulfilled: she had her own home to decorate, to invite friends and family to, and to bring up her children in. House and family, John and Marcia recalled, had always been the focal points of their mother's life. Church and assorted women's clubs had mattered, but not a great deal.

When John and then Marcia left home, first to go to college and then to get married, Sylvia had felt lost, abandoned. Her relationship with her husband, the children felt, was caring and dutiful but not precisely loving. Sylvia had increasingly come to depend on him in the years before he died. She had even, although reluctantly, let him help out around the house, though she continued to rule supreme in the kitchen. After her husband's death, Sylvia had been sad but not morbidly gloomy: she missed his company. She also missed the help he had provided, and John and Marcia had had to coax her to allow a housekeeper in once a week. But she continued to live independently, without involvement of community agencies such as the Visiting Nurse Association or the local senior center. The main joy in her life, as always, was her children—and now her two grandchildren as well.

While Nancy Kingsley talked to Sylvia's family, I conducted the physical examination. It was as revealing for what I did not find as for what I discovered. I did not find mild arm or leg weakness or impaired sensation to suggest an old stroke. I did not find the slow pulse and delayed reflexes characteristic of an underactive thyroid gland, which can produce cognitive and behavioral changes. Nor did I find the pattern of abnormal sensation in the legs characteristic of neuropathy, a condition that is often present with B_{12} deficiency and in some diabetics and alcoholics—and which can affect thinking as well.

The exam did yield two important findings. First, I discovered that while Mrs. Truman's exterior was immaculate, her personal hygiene was wanting. When she had removed her many layers of clothing, including a frayed and grayish girdle, stockings with runs, and soiled underwear, I found she badly needed a bath. Only a fairly significant neurologic deficit or a major depression could create the degree of apathy or lack of awareness necessary to allow so proud a woman as Sylvia Truman to let herself go. Second, I concluded the evaluation with a short mental status examination. "I'd like to see how your memory is," I said. "These are just routine questions, all right?" She nodded. "Did they tell you the name of this place?"

"General Hospital." Close, I thought.

"Do you know what year it is?"

"Nineteen—" She broke off, unsure.

"How about the month?" That she had no trouble with. "How about the day of the week?" That she knew too. "I'm going to give you three words to remember. I want you to store them away, and I'm going to ask you to tell me the words in a few minutes." Sylvia struggled to learn the three words, and in five minutes, when I asked her to recite them back to me, they were gone. She had no trouble with naming a few commonplace objects such as glasses and a watch, which gave the misleading impression that this skill was intact. My questions to her were too easy. She was able to write a grammatically correct sentence, when asked, but she chose "I am fine," which was not very demanding. Drawing a clock face with all the numbers and copying a simple diagram, two standard tests of visuo-spatial skill, were totally beyond her. She drew a circle that was far too small to accommodate the necessary numbers and then proceeded to put the numbers outside the circle, at first following the arc of her clock, but then abruptly proceeding horizontally. When copying my two intersecting pentagons, she seemed unable to perceive the overall geometric arrangement: she concentrated on each line segment individually, quickly losing track of their relationship to the whole. Her score, calculated by adding a point for each correct answer, was 20 out of a total possible 30.[1]

In the next stage of the assessment, the nurse practitioner, Joan Martin, gathered information about Mrs. Truman's "activities of daily living": her ability to dress herself, feed herself, wash herself, and perform such moderately more sophisticated chores as cooking and shopping. Her assessment included both reports from family members and direct observation of Mrs. Truman—as she got dressed after my exam, for instance. While she quizzed Sylvia's relatives, the team psychiatrist, who specialized in the care of the elderly, Dr. Samuel Jordan, performed more elaborate tests of mood and memory.

Nancy Kingsley, Joan Martin, Samuel Jordan, and I conferred briefly to share one another's findings. We had each gathered a few more clues—I with the mini-mental status exam, Joan with the revelation that burned pots had been found in Mrs. Truman's kitchen, Dr. Jordan with the history that Sylvia had never been depressed in her life and did not seem to be currently. Nancy had heard about the family's fears and their speculations. They were worried about putting Mrs. Truman in a nursing home, something they desperately wished to avoid. But they were worried about her safety at home, too, and in particular about her safety driving. As to their thoughts about what was wrong with her, they also did not believe she was depressed. She had never been the sort of person to be discouraged, let alone depressed. She had always taken life's vicissitudes in stride. She had been the pillar of strength who had held everything together when discord or misfortune threatened the family's stability. It would be out of character for her to be depressed. What they thought might be wrong with her—though they hoped they were mistaken— what they were afraid of and could hardly bring themselves to say, was that perhaps she had what her sister had had, at least what they were reasonably sure she had died of, though her doctor had never come out and said it—they had read about it in the newspapers—Alzheimer's disease.

Nancy and I went back into my office, where Mrs. Truman and her family had resumed their previous positions. Sylvia Truman looked tired. The consultation had lasted more than two hours so far, and she clearly had had enough. She was gazing out the window and could barely pay attention when I began speaking. Her family, on the other hand, were on tenterhooks. They were far more anxious than they had been earlier. Initially, they had been eager to unburden themselves, to tell us exactly what had been going on. They had wanted to be heard, to be certain we appreciated what they had been going through. But now they were awaiting the verdict, and they anticipated the worst.

I decided to begin with the positives. "You're basically a healthy woman," I told Sylvia, tapping her arm gently to attract her attention. "Physically you seem a lot younger than eighty-two." She looked pleased. The appeal to her vanity seemed like a good approach. "Really your main problem is your memory and more generally your thinking." She began to seem a bit apprehensive. "But that's nothing new to you, is it? You already know that you are sometimes forgetful and that your children have to remind you of appointments, of birthdays, of names." I tried to defuse the news by suggesting that all that had transpired in the preceding hours was that I now knew what she already knew about herself.

Mrs. Truman was moderately appeased by my strategy, but slightly suspicious, a tad defensive. "Everybody forgets things. Especially when you get to be my age. I don't think my memory's a problem. You should see some of my friends."

Of course it was entirely possible that her friends were worse off than she was. "You're right: memory problems are common as people get older. But your memory troubles are a little more than what I can attribute to normal aging. And your difficulties aren't just remembering—you have some trouble figuring out how to find your way around, and you're not as good at expressing yourself or doing arithmetic as I suspect you used to be." Sylvia Truman was not impressed by my attempt at flattery: she glared at me with hostility at the suggestion that she was not just as sharp as she had always been. John and Cynthia, whom I could see out of the corners of my eyes, looked as though they were about to leap out of their seats to protect Sylvia should my comments prove excessively threatening.

I decided I had delivered about as much bad news on one day as I could. Moreover, the diagnosis of dementia depended on excluding assorted reversible biochemical and structural brain abnormalities. The diagnosis of Alzheimer's disease required, in addition, progression over time. I could not, in good conscience, make a diagnosis at a single point in time. "There are a number of things that might be causing the memory difficulties, things that we can do something about. Medications can sometimes be the source of the problem, so I would like to be sure you stay off Elavil (the antidepressant) and Halcion (the sleeping pill)." I turned to Sylvia's children. "You should probably go through the medicine cabinet and throw out everything other than Tylenol and the blood pressure pills. In particular, make sure the Elavil and Halcion are discarded." They relaxed a little. This was something they could do. "I would also like to check a few blood tests to be sure your thyroid gland isn't out of whack and your B_{12} level is all right. A number of biochemical abnormalities can cause or worsen memory and judgment." I was addressing the entire Truman family now. I had lost Sylvia. She was looking over my head at the pictures on the wall. "Finally, I think we should get a CAT scan, a special X ray of the brain. Occasionally we find a collection of blood around the brain from a fall, or we diagnose a tumor. I doubt very much that you have anything like that, but if you did, we might be able to fix it, and I think it's important that we look for things we can do something about. In a month, after you've had all the tests, I'd like to see you back again." The atmosphere lightened measurably. The Truman family sensed that I was finished; I was ordering tests, none of which was objectionably invasive. While I had come alarmingly close to saying what they weren't sure they were ready to hear (and what they didn't want Sylvia to hear), I had managed to be both vague and honest.

"Is there anything else we should worry about right away?" Marcia wanted to know. "Should we be doing anything different?" The nurse practitioner answered by talking about safety issues: about checking whether Sylvia was burning pots or leaving the stove on and whether she was taking her blood pressure pills correctly. She promised to set up a home visit to look personally into other safety factors—whether the lighting was adequate and whether the house was cluttered, which would put Sylvia at risk for tripping and falling.

"Anything else on your minds?" the social worker inquired. The room was silent.

"Okay, Mom," John belted out as they all began extricating themselves from the crammed room. "Time for ice cream!" His mother brightened. The afternoon would be redeemed after all.

John escorted his mother to my secretary to schedule the CAT scan, point them in the direction of the lab where the blood work would be done, and schedule a follow-up appointment. Marcia, who had evidently established a good rapport with the social worker during their meeting, said an effusive good-bye to Nancy. Cynthia practically twitched with nervousness and lingered in my office after the others had proceeded to the waiting room. "There's one thing, Doctor," she began. Was she going to reveal some crucial bit of information, like the patient who spent the entire visit discussing chest pain, only to reveal on the way out the door that his real concern was that he might have AIDS? Or did she have a particular concern that she had been too shy to articulate in front of her family: was she perhaps worried that whatever her mother-in-law had was genetic and that her husband, too, was destined to get it? "We, I—after you get the tests back, when Sylvia comes in again, if it's Alzheimer's, I don't want you to tell her."

So that was it. Twenty-five years ago, American physicians had not told their patients if they had cancer. They told their families but kept the diagnosis a secret from their patients out of misguided paternalism. The physicians believed that if their patients knew they had a malignancy, they would become hopelessly depressed, possibly even suicidal. What they failed to recognize was that many if not most of their patients guessed the truth. Only the most naive patients dutifully went to the hospital three times a week for radiation therapy, or took medication that made them vomit and caused their hair to fall out, without suspecting they had cancer. Others fantasized about what was wrong with them, imagining diseases even worse than what they had. And many became angry at their betrayal by their physician and families, and fearful of further abandonment if they became sicker. Moreover, while many people were appropriately saddened by the disclosure of their cancer, few became clinically depressed, and only very, very rarely did a patient commit suicide. As a result of these observations, and with the developing support for patient autonomy by bioethicists, physicians began to tell their patients the truth.[2]

Physicians today are pretty good about revealing a cancer diagnosis. They are less good with other diseases, such as cirrhosis (in which the liver shrivels up) or cardiomyopathy (a degeneration of the heart muscle). When physicians do tell patients the name of their disease, they often fail to explain what it means, what the course of the illness is likely to be, and what the prognosis is. Dementia is today what cancer was a quarter of a century ago: a diagnosis shrouded in euphemism. Hadn't I been less than forthright, using terms such as "memory trouble" and "biochemical abnormalities"? But perhaps dementia is different from cancer or cirrhosis or cardiomyopathy. After all, by definition, many of the patients on whom I consulted who prove to have dementia, whether Alzheimer's disease or another variant of dementia, are incapable of understanding their diagnosis. No matter how simply I try to explain the problem, they do not have the intellectual capacity to process the significance of a progressive, relentless disturbance of cognitive function. The advanced cases are the easy ones. In those situations, I feel justified in confining my remarks to the family. Or if the patient is present, I can be sure the discussion is going over his head. If the patient did hear and understand a little bit, but the memory impairment was profound, he would recall nothing about the diagnosis a day later.

What about fairly mild, relatively early dementia—what Sylvia Truman had, if indeed she was demented? The major argument for informing patients that they have dementia is identical to the argument for explaining that they have any other medical disorder: only if individuals are knowledgeable about their minds and their bodies can they choose how to conduct their lives. A person with early Alzheimer's disease might live life very differently if he knew his diagnosis. If he were planning to move to a life care community—a retirement home—he might choose one with a nursing home on the premises, in anticipation of possibly requiring its services in the near future. He might be motivated to complete an advance directive, specifying what kinds of medical care he would or would not want in the future, and to appoint a family member as his health care proxy, empowered to make medical decisions on his behalf when he no longer could understand the issues himself. He might decide not to postpone that trip to Paris any longer, since he could still enjoy French cuisine and a trip to the Louvre but was less likely to be able to in a year or two.[3]

There is one well-publicized case of a woman who committed suicide after learning that she had Alzheimer's disease. She procured the services of Dr. Jack Kevorkian, who offered assisted suicide for just this sort of problem. The woman traveled from her home state of Oregon, where physician-assisted suicide was illegal, to Michigan, where it was not. She had a rendezvous with Dr. Kevorkian, and in a van containing his "suicide machine" pushed the button that triggered the release of the sedative thiopental, followed automatically by a lethal dose of potassium. At the time of her death, she was described as having word-finding and reading-comprehension problems interfering with her ability to work as a teacher and to play the piano. She was able to play tennis and was reported to enjoy her family life.[4]

The fact that an occasional patient with early Alzheimer's disease who knows her diagnosis commits suicide does not imply that patients should never be told the truth. Some patients with Alzheimer's disease who are *not* told their diagnosis also commit suicide. The number of suicides can be expected to be small, both because people in general do not kill themselves over a diagnosis, as was found with cancer patients, and because individuals with dementia have particular difficulty designing and executing a new and complex plan.

The most compelling argument against telling a patient he has dementia is that individuals with dementia already have impaired autonomy *because* of their dementia, and therefore knowing their diagnosis will not permit them to exercise their autonomy. Thus, the only possible consequence of disclosure, the argument goes, is depression or suicidal thoughts, without the compensatory benefit of heightened autonomy. The counterargument is that while patients with dementia have diminished autonomy in the early stages, they have not completely lost their ability to exercise self-determination. Knowledge of their diagnosis allows them to make some of the few choices they can still make. What counts at least as much as *whether* to tell is *how* to tell. How the physician reveals the diagnosis must vary depending on the patient's ability to understand. Just as a patient with cancer does not necessarily need to be told the trajectory, the life expectancy, all possible treatments and each of their likely outcomes at the first office visit, so, too, the patient with dementia does not have to be hit over the head with the whole truth and nothing but the truth.

That's more or less what I told Cynthia as she shifted her bag anxiously from one shoulder to the other. "I don't think we can hide the truth from your mother-in-law. And I don't think she would want us to conceal anything from her. But if she does have a progressive dementia, I can talk about it very matter-of-factly. I won't take a deep breath and announce in a solemn voice that she has Alzheimer's. I can say quite casually that there is evidence of what we call dementia, and this is what we should do about it." Cynthia looked skeptical. "I guess you have experience with this sort of thing," she said, "but I just don't want you to hurt my mother-in-law. She's been like a mother to me."

"I understand," I told her. "You wish you could protect her from being sick. I wish I could cure this thing—let's hope one of the tests is positive so I'll have something to treat. But even if Sylvia doesn't have thyroid disease or B_{12} deficiency to explain some of her symptoms, there are things we can do to help. Lying to her, at this point, isn't one of them." Cynthia nodded and joined the rest of her family.

One month later, John Truman brought his mother back for her follow-up appointment. This time he came without his wife and sister. John was his usual jovial self, and Sylvia was her usual well-dressed but remote self. "How are things?" I asked. "About the same," John told me. Sylvia said nothing. "Did you have a chance to get rid of the medications we discussed?" I asked as I read over my notes from the initial consultation. "Did we ever! We found some amazing stuff in your bathroom, didn't we, Mom? Pills from ten years ago. Three different kinds of blood pressure medication. We had a field day cleaning everything up." John was so cheerful that his mother smiled, too, but I could not determine whether his ebullience was infectious or whether she actually recalled with amusement the purging of her medicine cabinet. "Do you think she'd been taking any of that stuff?" I wondered out loud. John turned to his mother. "You didn't take any of those old pills, did you, Mom?" She shrugged her shoulders. "I don't think so," he continued. "I don't think she's been taking *any* medications, new or old. We had a hard time finding the bottle of the stuff she's supposed to be taking. And most of the old medicines were off in the downstairs bathroom, which Mom hardly ever uses. But it was a good idea to clean everything up. Wouldn't want the mice to get poisoned on that outdated stuff." Sylvia looked alarmed. "It's okay, Mom. There are no mice. I was just joking. I don't think disposing of the old pills had any effect on the memory, but it was a good move anyway."

He had brought up the memory problem, so I had my entree to the main topic for today: Sylvia Truman's test results and what they indicated about her mental status. I told the two of them that I had received all the reports, and they showed that Mrs. Truman was remarkably healthy. She was not anemic. Her thyroid tests, her liver tests, and her other blood chemistries were all perfectly normal. Her CAT scan showed moderate atrophy, or shrinkage, of brain tissue, which was consistent with her age and not diagnostic of any disease. At this point in the litany, I saw that I had already lost Sylvia's attention. She was staring out the window. I shifted slightly in my seat so that I was facing John more directly, since he was the one who was listening. I explained that there were no tumors or collections of blood or small strokes on the CAT scan. Given Mrs. Truman's cognitive impairment—both by history and from the testing that I had performed—and the lack of any acute illness that might transiently render her confused, I felt she had what we called dementia. Dementia, I went on, was a wastebasket term for a variety of disorders. In all of them, the affected individual had losses in several domains of mental functioning, typically memory and several others such as language, visuo-spatial orientation, and judgment. Sylvia's inability to copy a simple figure I had drawn on a sheet of paper indicated a deficit in visuo-spatial skills. In real life, the episode in which she wandered around looking for her house probably occurred in part because of problems with orientation in three-dimensional space. It also reflected a deficit in judgment, since she should have realized that she couldn't get in the door because she had forgotten her keys, not because she was at the wrong house. Sylvia's sometimes comical use of words—her calling a teaspoon a "scoop" or a "ladle" and her corresponding difficulty in telling me the name of an object I showed her during the testing—arose from a flaw in her ability to use language.

John was following everything I said. He seemed to grasp what I meant by dementia. "You said there are different kinds of dementia. Can you tell from the tests which kind she has?" In response, I continued my explanation. "The most common form of dementia is Alzheimer's disease. The next most common form is multi-infarct dementia, which is due to many small strokes, sometimes strokes the patient may be unaware of, that cumulatively destroy enough brain cells in particular places so as to produce dementia. Then there are a number of potentially reversible causes of dementia: gland problems, such as an underactive thyroid or an overactive parathyroid gland. Those are the things I was looking for with the blood tests. Other treatable dementias are those due to physical problems in the brain, things we talked about, such as a subdural hematoma, a collection of blood between the skull and the brain that can result from a fall. The tests your mother had demonstrate that she doesn't have any of the possibly curable types of dementia. Her CAT scan does not show any old strokes, there's nothing on my exam to suggest she's had strokes in the past, and none of you remember times when she had trouble with her arms or legs or talking or seeing, do you?" I looked to John for confirmation. He shook his head. "It's *conceivable* your mother did have a series of small strokes—she does have high blood pressure so she certainly is at risk for strokes—and an MRI would be better than a CAT scan for picking up subtle changes."

For the first time in this recitation, John seemed irritated. "So why didn't you order an MRI? Or are you going to want to put her through another test now?"

I told him about the MRI scanner—how the patient had to lie motionless in a confined, tunnel-like machine for half an hour, and how when the giant magnet was turned on, it made sounds like a jackhammer. Modern CAT scanning, by contrast, was quick and quiet. The grin returned to John's face. He agreed that his mother would be terrified by an MRI. The CAT scan had been bad enough. He shared my view that the more sophisticated test was not warranted solely to permit making what at this point was the academic distinction between Alzheimer's disease and multi-infarct dementia. The CAT scan had been adequate to exclude an accumulation of blood under the skull, a tumor, and other potentially treatable disorders such as normal pressure hydrocephalus, a condition in which the fluid that normally cushions the brain does not circulate properly, builds up, and causes, among other problems, dementia.

"So you're saying she has Alzheimer's," John finished for me.

"Probably. There is no definitive test for Alzheimer's short of a brain biopsy. It's a diagnosis of exclusion—if someone has dementia, and all other causes have been eliminated, then it's most likely Alzheimer's. To fit the definition of Alzheimer's, the disorder must be progressive. So I'll want to see your mom in another six months, and I think then we can be a little more certain."[5]

I wasn't sure how much more John wanted to hear today. Sylvia was getting bored—her eyes were closing. I tapped her hand quietly to draw her in. "We've been talking about your memory problem." Her eyes were open now. "There are no special medications for this. In fact, one of the major treatments is to avoid any medications that could make things worse. And not just prescription medicines—over-the-counter drugs, too: things like cold preparations, particularly antihistamines. And something else to avoid is alcohol. Do you drink?" Sylvia and John both laughed. Evidently Sylvia drank a glass of champagne on New Year's Eve and that was about it.

"At this point, when your memory troubles are not very severe, my main concern is just to make sure you have whatever help you need to be as independent as possible—and as safe as possible."

Right on cue, John piped up. "What about her driving, Doctor?"

The issue of driving and dementia is not nearly as straight-forward as one might think. Nor, for that matter, is the subject of driving and the overall elderly population clear-cut. What is known is that drivers over age sixty-five do not have any more reported accidents per driver per year than drivers under sixty-five—though they have far more accidents *per mile*. Elderly drivers are correct when they report that they do not drive much and that they mainly drive in their own neighborhoods. When their short trips are taken into consideration, what becomes evident is that accidents per mile rise steadily with the age of the driver after sixty-five. While it's true that fatalities are likely to be higher if a crash occurs on the highway than if it takes place on city streets, simply because the driver's velocity is usually greater, crashes in the neighborhood can also be devastating. For one thing, they are far more likely to involve pedestrians. Though there is no threshold age above which drivers suddenly become unsafe, driving skills deserve careful assessment, on an individual basis, as people age.

Elderly drivers with declining mental capacity are a sub-group whose driving skills are particularly in need of evaluation. Unfortunately, there is no direct correlation between the degree of cognitive impairment—as determined, for instance, by the score on a mental status examination—and the degree of driving impairment. Many older people with mild dementia get by without any automobile accidents. To deprive them of the freedom afforded by being able to drive does not seem justified simply on the commonsense theory that people with memory problems, judgment problems, or visuo-spatial difficulties are hazardous on the road. At some point in their illness, individuals with dementia unambiguously cannot drive safely. But as yet there are no tests that clearly demarcate the safe drivers with dementia from those who are unsafe.[6]

One promising means of testing driver safety is a simulated road test. Such tests are available in some areas and serve to point out problem areas to drivers. Ideally, test subjects who experience difficulty with left turns or dealing with detour signs or making sudden stops will themselves recognize that if they have trouble behind a mock steering wheel they should not be driving behind a real one. Such assessments, however, are not universally available, they tend to be expensive, and those drivers whose judgment has been impaired by dementia may not draw the appropriate conclusions from the test.

The only unequivocally good predictor of future accidents is previous accidents. Anyone who has dementia and who has been responsible for a car accident is at risk of causing future accidents and should stop driving. Actually inducing an individual to give up his or her car is another hurdle. The Bureau of Motor Vehicles does not routinely check mental status, in part because of the poor correlation between any single measure of cognitive ability and driving capacity. Physicians can, in some states, prevent the renewal of a driver's license with a firmly worded letter to the authorities. An alternative strategy is for families to allow their impaired relative to keep the car, but either to disable the car or to permanently hide the car keys. Such subterfuge, like concealing the diagnosis of dementia, usually creates frustration rather than a satisfactory resolution of a painful dilemma. Unfortunately, deception is sometimes the only way simultaneously to save face and save lives.

I hoped to be able to cajole Sylvia Truman into forgoing driving without resorting to deception. "I only drive near my house and I don't go out at night," she asserted, as though that proved her competence.

"But Mom," John protested. "Do you remember how many times you've had the car in the shop in the last six months? I think it's been at the mechanic's as much as it's been in your garage."

"It's not my fault Joe is so slow with the repairs. And I didn't cause any accidents," Mrs. Truman maintained defensively.

"Aw, Mom, come on! When you swerved off the road and hit a tree, was it the tree's fault?" We all laughed, but Sylvia quickly resumed her hostile stance. "I haven't had any more accidents than anyone else I know. And I don't see how I can get by without a car. How will I go do my shopping or go visiting?"

Therein lay the crux of the problem. It also contained the key to the solution. Like the vast majority of suburban or rural Americans, Sylvia Truman did not live in walking distance of all her friends or her favorite shops, nor could she reach them by public transportation. Even if bus or trolley routes had existed covering the requisite terrain, Sylvia's arthritic knees, while generally adequate for her daily activities, would not have been up to the task of boarding a bus. In fact, while the rest of the world might have been a tiny bit safer had Sylvia Truman substituted public for private transportation, her personal safety might be further jeopardized as she tried to cross broad streets or stood, unsupported, on a swaying trolley car.

The alternative to her own car could not be a bus or subway; it had to be someone else's car. Brazenly, I asked Sylvia, with her son's assistance, to compute the annual cost of her car's upkeep. How much did she spend on routine maintenance, on gasoline, on insurance (an astronomical sum, if she reported her accidents), and on repairs? A rough calculation revealed that she spent at least $3,000 a year on her car. "Three thousand a year," I suggested, "can pay for an awful lot of taxi rides." John beamed. He promised to obtain the telephone number of a reliable cab company. I indicated that there were a few companies that offered a discount to senior citizens. Sylvia liked the idea of a bargain. She promised to think about my proposal.

The other major safety issue had been addressed by Nancy Kingsley, the social worker. She had been concerned about Sylvia's ability to cook and shop for herself after learning about the burned pots. She had followed up with Cynthia, who seemed to be in charge of Sylvia's domestic affairs. Cynthia reported that she had checked her mother-in-law's refrigerator and had discovered an assortment of fungi living on the few withered pieces of fruit and hunks of cheese. She had been shocked by how bare the refrigerator was: a few cans of soda, half a loaf of slightly stale bread, a jar of pickles, a container of cottage cheese, and some marmalade. The cupboards were only marginally more promising: plenty of tea bags, cans of soup, a box of cereal, and a large supply of instant rice. The freezer was filled with ready-made microwavable dinners, all of which contained protein and some of which boasted a portion of vegetables. Cynthia had already hired a housekeeper to come in three days a week to do some cleaning and buy supplies. Nancy hooked her up with the local Meals on Wheels program, so Sylvia could get a hot meal five days a week. The two children decided to split the weekends—one weekend Marcia would take her mother to her house, provide some social stimulation, three square meals a day, and a bath; the following weekend John would take over. So far, there had been no more wandering incidents. They hoped that with the housekeeper and the home-delivered meals, Sylvia would have little occasion to cook, thereby minimizing the risk of a fire. Fortunately, she did not smoke. Eventually she would need greater supervision; for the time being, the arrangement sufficed.

Before the Trumans left the office, John wanted to be sure there wasn't anything else he needed to attend to immediately. A discussion of what the future held in store could wait, at least until the six-month follow-up visit, at which time I would be even more certain regarding the diagnosis. There was one matter worth dealing with right away, and that was designating a health care proxy. The Trumans might wish to postpone thinking about how much or what kind of medical care would be appropriate for Sylvia if she became acutely ill, but the problem was that if she got sick she would be even less capable than she was now of participating in decisions about her care. Now, while she was physically healthy, her mind operating on only three cylinders but working well enough to recognize and communicate with her family, she could identify whom she wanted to serve as decision maker for her, if necessary. I explained that her primary care doctor would discuss any problems with her if they arose. She would always be able to say she did or did not want some medical procedure that her doctor thought might help her—or might help him figure out what was wrong—provided she was able to understand the pros and cons of the procedure. "Sometimes," I said gingerly, "when people are sick, the oxygen in their blood is very low or their temperature is very high, or there are noxious chemicals in their system, any of which can make it hard for them to think straight." I added, by way of clarification to John, that this sort of confusion could happen to anyone, though the elderly were especially prone to it, and the demented elderly even more susceptible. "So it's not a bad idea for everyone to choose a health care proxy, to pick one person—usually but not necessarily a relative—to serve as his spokesperson, just in case."

I turned back to Sylvia. "Is there someone you would want your doctor to talk to about your medical problems if you were very sick and decisions needed to be made for you, which you couldn't make yourself? One of your children perhaps?"

Sylvia looked a little puzzled. "John, I guess. He's the lawyer." I assured her that she did not need a lawyer to serve as her surrogate—and she did not even need a lawyer to draw up the necessary papers: I had a stack of forms for designating a health care proxy in my desk drawer. "It would make Marcia too nervous," Sylvia continued insightfully. "It would give her nightmares. And Cynthia is like a daughter to me, but she isn't my blood. So I guess the job falls to John after all. Being a lawyer doesn't disqualify him, does it?" I was pleased to see that Sylvia could still be witty. "No," I assured her, "he can be your proxy if you're sure you want him." I handed John a copy of a form that was compatible with the Massachusetts health care proxy statute and urged them to complete it at home. The form required two witnesses and allowed for selection of an alternate proxy if John proved unavailable at the crucial moment. The version I used also had a section in which the patient or potential patient could specify particular preferences. She might, for instance, state categorically that if her heart stopped she would not wish to be resuscitated. She might choose to spell out that if she were irreversibly comatose, she would not wish her life prolonged with artificial nutrition. I was not convinced that Sylvia could fully grasp the implication of such choices, but thought she and her newly selected health care proxy should try to discuss them. Finally, I emphasized the importance of giving a copy of the completed document to Sylvia's primary care physician. All too many individuals dutifully choose a proxy, write down reams about their desires if they became critically ill, and then lock the advance directive in a safe deposit box.

I exhorted John to keep in touch if there were new developments. I indicated that Sylvia's regular doctor should handle any medical problems that arose. I would send him a letter summarizing my findings and we would get together in another six months.

CHAPTER 2

Alzheimer's Disease—
the Science

Until just a few years ago, physicians did not need to know very much about the scientific underpinnings of Alzheimer's disease. Patients, families, and the general public had little reason to be concerned with the scant anatomic and biochemical details. If a practicing physician for some reason wanted to learn about the science, there was not terribly much to know. The hallmarks of the disease were plaques and tangles: plaques are proteinaceous deposits outside cells and neurofibrillary tangles are the debris inside neurons, both described by Alois Alzheimer in the beginning of the twentieth century. Plaques and tangles could be counted more accurately and described more precisely in 1986 than in 1906, thanks to new technology, but Alzheimer's disease research was still primarily descriptive rather than mechanistic; it centered on detailing *what* happened to a person's brain cells and to his behavior rather than *how* or *why* it happened.

All this has changed dramatically over the past ten years. Research on Alzheimer's has grown exponentially. Even general medical journals, which prior to 1994 only very occasionally featured a study on Alzheimer's—and then it was typically an epidemiologic study, measuring the pervasiveness of cognitive impairment in the population—began to publish several articles each year on the basic science of dementia.[1] Familiarity with the science has suddenly become important. It is important first as a backdrop to recruiting patients into clinical trials—studies testing the ability of medications to delay the onset of the progression of Alzheimer's. At the same time, it is critical to understand the science in order to grasp the limitations of those trials and hence to realize that although tremendous progress is being made, a cure is *not* just around the corner.

The story of Alzheimer's research over the last decade opens a window onto biomedical research in general. It reveals with stunning clarity what factors—technical, intellectual, and political—fuel the engine of American science.

In the Beginning

When Alois Alzheimer (1864–1915) was a physician working at a mental institution in Frankfurt, Germany, he was in charge of the case of Frau Auguste D. At age fifty-one, Mrs. D. had trouble with her memory, frequently could not find the words to express herself, and began having difficulty figuring out how to perform such everyday tasks as dressing herself or combing her hair. After admission to the asylum, she progressively deteriorated. By the time of her death at age fifty-five, Frau D. was incontinent and spent her days lying curled up in a fetal position. Alzheimer, who was by training a neuropathologist, performed an autopsy and found a small, shrunken brain. When he used a special silver stain to visualize the cells of the cerebral cortex, the part of the brain responsible for thinking, he found dense bundles of fibrils where the nerve cells had once been. Alzheimer concluded that these "neurofibrillary tangles," which had not previously been described, were the essential feature of Mrs. D.'s dementia. Alzheimer also noted that, spread over the entire cortex, was a "peculiar substance" designated by others as plaques. Much of the science of Alzheimer's has consisted of unraveling the mysteries of tangles and plaques, identified years later as containing the proteins tau and amyloid respectively.

The Amyloid Story

Alzheimer's finding of plaques in the brain of Frau Auguste D. was soon duplicated by other scientists. Pathologists had earlier noticed plaques in the brains of older individuals diagnosed with "senility"; Alzheimer's contribution was to find the same material present in younger patients diagnosed with a "presenile" form of dementia. What plaques were made of, how they got into the brain, and whether they caused disease were unknown. Without any new techniques for studying plaques, and given a whole slew of other more readily soluble medical problems, their nature remained a mystery for decades. In the 1930s, a Belgian pathologist discovered a clue to the identity of the "peculiar substance" described by Alzheimer in the brains of demented individuals—it took up stains just like amyloid, a protein that was known to cause a whole host of problems when it accumulated in excessive amounts in a variety of organs.[2] Then, in 1964, the neurologist Robert Terry decided to examine brain specimens from patients diagnosed as having Alzheimer's disease using the electron microscope. Terry demonstrated that plaques "have as their fundamental substance . . . a filamentous material which is structurally identical to amyloid."[3] This substance differed from what he found in tangles. In the immediate vicinity of the amyloid were microglia, scavenger cells, which "seemed to be the source of the amyloid," but the association was due to proximity alone.

The static, photographic view of the brain that Terry obtained could not answer the question of what role amyloid played. It was possible that amyloid was not involved in dementia at all—either as cause or effect—but was simply a concomitant of normal aging. Nonetheless, several research groups in different parts of the world, including Australia, Germany, and the United States, gambled that amyloid was the key to Alzheimer's disease. By the mid-1980s, using sophisticated biochemical analysis, the amyloid core of plaques had been more precisely characterized: it was a small protein folded in a particular three-dimensional pattern called a beta-pleated sheet. The small protein soon yielded its complete identity to scientists—it is a chain of between thirty-nine and forty-two amino acids. This same sequence was found not only in the cerebral cortex of Alzheimer's patients but also lining their blood vessels and the meninges, the filmy cover of the brain and spinal cord.

Scientists found that the small beta-amyloid peptide was

derived from a larger, 695–amino acid protein. Frequently, important body chemicals such as insulin or thyroid hormone are literally cut out of bigger precursor molecules. This allows for storage of a large amount of inactive material that can quickly be converted into the needed substance on demand—since the limiting factor in the assembly process is gathering the raw materials. Beta-amyloid turned out to be cleaved from the beta-amyloid precursor protein (APP). Normally, the precursor protein is cut in such a way that the by-products do not include beta-amyloid. Sometimes, particularly in individuals with Alzheimer's disease, the precursor protein is split so that beta-amyloid is produced.

As a result of the work on the biochemistry of amyloid, we now have more than a mere description of diseased brains; we have an intriguing hypothesis about the pathophysiology of the disorder—what goes wrong and how the flaw injures brain tissue. Understanding the sequence of events that appear to lead up to Alzheimer's opens the way to possible modes of diagnosis and treatment. If amyloid is the root cause of Alzheimer's disease, then research investigating what stimulates the abnormal deposition of amyloid and elucidating the exact biochemical steps whereby amyloid causes problems could lead to cure. Chemicals that protect neurons, called nootropic agents, are actively under investigation—an approach that is analogous to protective masks for miners exposed to toxic fumes. Alternatively, if all the steps in the "cascade" leading to amyloid-mediated nerve death are identified, then conceivably a drug could be custom designed to interfere with one crucial step, and amyloid would not be manufactured in the first place.

Though countless studies have correlated amyloid with Alzheimer's, the possibility remains that amyloid is a product of dying nerve cells, rather like the enzyme creatine phosphokinase (CPK) released by dying heart muscle that allows physicians to diagnose a heart attack. The CPK elevation is clearly not the *cause* of a myocardial infarction; it is the by-product of tissue death. The fact that all old people develop some amyloid deposits in their brains, and that the level rises with increasing age, even in those with no signs of dementia, suggests that amyloid may not have a primary role in causing Alzheimer's.

Surely the question of which comes first, amyloid or nerve-death, should be easy to answer. Studies have been done confirming that when nerve cells are cultured in a petri dish, and amyloid is added, the nerve cells die. However, this sort of artificial, test tube experiment does not prove that the same thing happens in the brain of a living animal. When Bruce Yankner in Boston injected amyloid into the brains of live rats, sacrificed the rats, and was able to show that plaques had developed at the injection sites, his results seemed definitive. Critics, however, attributed the reaction to the injection itself, claiming it had nothing to do with *what* was injected, and everything to do with the *process* of injection. Researchers at other labs who tried to duplicate Yankner's work were unable to do so. Frustrated that months and in some cases years of work had gone down the drain, they attacked him for allegedly being "uncooperative" in sharing information about his methods. Other researchers acknowledged that Yankner had been quite forthcoming about the technical aspects of his work, and indicated they were put off by his brash assertions that his work constituted a major breakthrough. However, scientists in their excitement are often immodest about their contributions, so it seems implausible to blame the intense hostility evoked by Yankner to a few ill-chosen remarks. At one of the annual Society for Neuroscience meetings, tempers were so high that Zaven Khachaturian, head of the Alzheimer's program at the National Institute on Aging, felt professional mediation might be necessary. The high financial and emotional stakes had escalated the conflict to new heights. Ultimately, the editors of the journal *Neurobiology of Aging* decided to devote an entire issue to papers addressing the question of amyloid's toxicity. While no clear consensus emerged from this special issue, it suggested an important role for amyloid, though it discounted Yankner's animal model findings.[4] The discovery that some cases of early-onset, familial Alzheimer's are due to a defect in the gene coding for the amyloid precursor protein is further evidence of a central role for amyloid. Given the persistent ambiguity surrounding amyloid, a rival camp has appeared, which believes the culprit is another protein entirely, the molecule called *tau*.

The Story of Tau

In reporting on the autopsy of Frau Auguste D., his first patient with "presenile dementia," Alois Alzheimer principally directed his attention to the "neurofibrillary tangles" inside brain cells. He also noted the presence of plaques, which had previously been described in the brains of older people with "senile dementia." Tangles were new and different. Using a special stain that he and his coworkers had invented, Alzheimer found that between one fourth and one third of the cortical neurons in Frau D.'s brain were reduced to dense, tangled bundles of neurofibrils. These looked like the skeletal remains of cells whose nuclei, or centers, had completely disintegrated. For fifty years, scientists learned little more about tangles than what Alzheimer had described: further analysis of tangles had to await the development of techniques more powerful than light microscopy.

When the electron microscope was turned on tangles in the 1960s, they were found to consist of pairs of helically twisted filaments (abbreviated PHFs). Researchers in the pathology department at Albert Einstein College of Medicine in New York City, using new biochemical and immunochemical techniques, discovered that a major ingredient of PHFs was the protein tau.

Tau, it turned out, has the job within the neuron of stabilizing microtubules, which are involved in ferrying nutrients from one part of the cell to another. When tau attaches to microtubules, they are structurally strong, able to carry their cargo. When tau does not bind properly to microtubules, they weaken and collapse. With its transport routes cut off, the cell cannot survive.

What goes wrong in Alzheimer's disease is that tau is chemically altered (by the addition of phosphorus-containing molecules) so that it no longer interacts properly with microtubules.[5] When nerve cells growing in a laboratory petri dish are deprived of tau, they undergo changes that are remarkably similar to the changes seen in neurons in Alzheimer's.[6]

The tau theory, like the amyloid theory, has dramatic implications both for diagnosis and for treatment. If the abnormal version of tau is unique to Alzheimer's disease (unlike amyloid, which is clearly found both in other disorders and in normal aging), then finding it in a person suspected of having Alzheimer's could clinch the diagnosis. So far, the only reliable means of finding tau in a living person is with a brain biopsy, which is not particularly practical. However, preliminary evidence suggests that tau can also be measured in the cerebrospinal fluid, the fluid lining the brain and spinal cord, which can be sampled with a lumbar puncture. Elevated levels are far more likely in Alzheimer's than in patients with other chronic neurologic diseases or in normal subjects.[7]

If tau is truly the key to Alzheimer's disease, then the disease could be prevented by finding a drug that selectively modifies the biochemical pathway whose end product is the abnormal form of tau. While this sounds farfetched, in fact scientists are successfully identifying these chemical reactions. Moreover, there is precedent for finding drugs that interfere with metabolism. We can prevent gout, for example, a condition due to excessive amounts of uric acid, with the drug allopurinol, which decreases uric acid production. Antibiotics typically work by taking advantage of the fact that bacterial metabolism and human metabolism differ—so as to be able to interfere selectively with a critical step in the production of a substance necessary for bacterial reproduction. The tricky aspect of targeting tau is finding a drug that can cross the "blood-brain barrier," the system of tightly linked capillaries designed to keep undesirable substances out of the central nervous system, and ensuring that the *only* reaction affected is the one involved in adding excessive numbers of phosphorus molecules to tau. If the reaction that is abnormal and to be avoided in the brain proves to be normal and necessary elsewhere in the body, chemical manipulation could have widespread and devastating effects. This is the basis of the toxicity of most cancer chemotherapy: agents are designed that are toxic to rapidly dividing cells on the grounds that cancer cells tend to be rapidly dividing. Unfortunately, normal skin cells and cells lining the intestines and bone marrow cells are also rapidly dividing and hence are often destroyed by chemotherapy.

In the search for the fundamental cause of Alzheimer's disease, tau and amyloid remain prime suspects. Other investigators, however, have been following a different lead: a brain chemical that is essential for *memory*.

The Acetylcholine Story

At just about the time Alzheimer made his critical discoveries in Germany, doctors in the United States were beginning to use a drug with powerful effects on memory. The drug was called scopolamine, and it was employed together with morphine to produce a new form of obstetric anesthesia, popularly known as "twilight sleep." The morphine was administered in small quantities to treat labor pains, and the scopolamine was used so women would forget they had had labor pains. Remarkable as it seems today, many vocal, upper-class women demanded this approach to labor and delivery, because even though the treatment often left them screaming in pain, necessitating the use of special "cribs" to restrain them as they thrashed, it also left them with no memory of the entire period of labor and delivery. They emerged "fresh and invigorated," blissfully unaware of the agony they had endured.[8]

The revolutionary feature of this technique for managing childbirth was the use of scopolamine. Scopolamine has been around for at least two thousand years. It is a belladonna alkaloid, so named for its ability to cause the pupils to dilate, a phenomenon thought to create a "beautiful woman." It is a first cousin of atropine, which in turn is derived from the poisonous nightshade plant. Nightshade was used during the Roman Empire to produce slow and insidious poisoning; the belladonna alkaloids in more modest doses were used by physicians for centuries to combat diarrhea. But though high doses of atropine cause irritability and hallucinations, atropine in lower doses cannot cross the "blood-brain barrier." Scopolamine acts in much the same way as atropine, but it gets into the brain itself.

Both atropine and scopolamine block the effects of acetylcholine, a chemical released by certain nerves in order to transmit messages to muscles and other nerves. Atropine's effects are largely confined to nerves in the peripheral nervous system: it can decrease salivation and sweating; in higher doses it causes the pupils to dilate and the heart rate to accelerate; in even larger doses it prevents the bladder from emptying and the intestines from contracting. Scopolamine does the same thing but it also affects the brain, with remarkable results: it can counteract motion sickness and can induce forgetfulness. Because scopolamine has a nasty tendency to cause confusion and agitation, even when given in the same dose that, on other occasions, causes euphoria, it fell out of favor. Alternative approaches to obstetric anesthesia were discovered. When blockage of acetylcholine was desired—for instance to treat a dangerously low heart rate or to control diarrhea—atropine was the preferred drug. Scopolamine's peculiar effects on memory lay forgotten, unstudied for half a century.

Then, in 1974, David Drachman and his colleagues at the Northwestern University School of Medicine published a remarkable study. They looked at the effects of scopolamine on memory in young, healthy people (students of various types) and compared the performance of the scopolamine-treated students on a variety of tests of memory to the performance of older people (volunteers aged fifty-nine to eighty-seven, with an average age of sixty-seven) on the same tests. What they found was that the young subjects given scopolamine developed difficulty with certain memory tests, in particular those involving the storage and retrieval of information beyond the limits of very short-term memory. On other tests of memory and cognition, the students had no difficulty, despite the scopolamine. The older volunteers, who got no medication, had impairment on exactly the same memory tests.[9] The results suggested that acetylcholine was critically involved with memory, and that the mild memory deficits commonly accompanying seemingly normal aging might be due to a failure of cholinergic (acetylcholine-producing) neurons.

If mild memory loss looked like a case of scopolamine poisoning, perhaps the more severe memory loss of Alzheimer's disease was due to a problem with cholinergic neurons, too. And indeed, two separate laboratories independently discovered that the brains of patients with Alzheimer's disease could be shown at autopsy to have a dramatic decrease in the number of cholinergic neurons. With this finding, a mere two years after Drachman's article was published, a new theory was born. Alzheimer's disease might be an acetylcholine deficiency disease, much as Parkinson's disease, another degenerative neurologic disorder, is due to deficiency of the brain biochemical dopamine.

Quantifying the magnitude of the loss of cholinergic neurons and mapping just which nerves are lost in Alzheimer's disease led to additional intriguing revelations. In advanced Alzheimer's, up to 90 percent of the acetylcholine content of the cortex (the part of the brain associated with thinking) is lost. The loss of acetylcholine activity is not evenly distributed throughout the brain—it happens to occur in just those areas of the brain associated with memory, such as the hippocampus.[10]

These observations generated tremendous excitement among neuroscientists because of their potential implications for treatment. If the memory and cognitive deficits of Alzheimer's disease are due to too little acetylcholine, then perhaps they can be overcome by acetylcholine replacement therapy. Unfortunately, administering oral acetylcholine itself is not clinically useful: it is destroyed within minutes of reaching the bloodstream. Its precursor, choline or lecithin, can, however, be given as a pill. Despite its promise as a therapeutic agent, lecithin simply does not work to enhance memory. One reason for this disappointing finding may be that older people's ability to transport dietary choline into the brain is limited—whether or not they have Alzheimer's disease.[11]

Instead of giving up on acetylcholine, some researchers set out to prevent destruction of the acetylcholine already present in the brain rather than to boost the supply. Acetylcholine is broken down in the body by a substance called acetylcholinesterase. Drugs that enter the brain and counteract acetylcholinesterase can be expected to increase the amount of acetylcholine in the brain. Perhaps surprisingly, a chemical that does exactly this occurs in nature in the Calibar bean. It was once used as an "ordeal poison" in trials for witchcraft: suspected witches were given the drug, and if they survived the hallucinations, palpitations, and high blood pressure it induced, they were presumed innocent. First purified in England in 1864 and given the scientific name physostigmine, it was found thirteen years later to be useful in treating glaucoma, an eye disease, a role it continues to have today. Scientists tried using physostigmine to improve the memory of normal individuals but were unsuccessful. While the drug showed some promise when used in Alzheimer's disease, its side effects—the same sort that made physostigmine popular in witch trials—limited its usefulness.

The temptation to treat Alzheimer's disease as acetylcholine deficiency remained very strong despite these initial failures. After all, other medical diseases that are characterized by deficient production of some critical bodily fluid have been successfully treated through replacement therapy. The insulin deficiency of diabetes, for example, can be overcome by insulin injections, and the missing thyroid hormone of hypothyroidism can be remedied through thyroxine pills. Replenishing a hormone circulating in the blood is considerably easier than restoring a brain chemical that is normally released by nerves when they fire. But the conviction that elevating acetylcholine in the brain *must* be helpful in Alzheimer's disease was the inspiration behind tacrine, the first drug approved by the Food and Drug Administration for use in Alzheimer's disease.

Tacrine, or tetrahydroaminoacridine, is an artificially created compound that works much like physostigmine. It inhibits breakdown of acetylcholine, thus raising the levels of the neurotransmitter. Unfortunately, tacrine has at best limited utility—it may improve test scores and day-to-day functioning for some individuals to a modest extent. At worst, it must be discontinued because of side effects: about two thirds of individuals taking the higher doses of the drug discontinue the medication, either because of nausea or, in nearly one third of cases, because of abnormalities in blood tests of liver function.[12] Some physicians argue that tacrine is simply a third-rate drug: it's expensive, it has side effects, and it scarcely works, if at all (see Chapter 6 on the politics of tacrine). Even its advocates acknowledge that tacrine is not the answer to Alzheimer's disease. But its development has shown that the acetylcholine piece of the Alzheimer's puzzle is a fruitful area for research. Donepezil (Aricept), a new tacrine-like drug that has fewer side effects, was approved by the Food and Drug Administration in 1996, and other pharmacological manipulations are in the works.

In the final analysis, it is not surprising that merely raising the quantity of acetylcholine in the brain should be inadequate to treat Alzheimer's disease. In many cases, the neurons that need the chemical have already died, so replacement therapy is far too late. More generally, acetylcholine is not like thyroid hormone—a substance that must be maintained in the circulation at fairly constant levels. It is packaged by nerve cells and released at nerve endings to send messages. To expect that stocking up on the biochemical will solve the problem is naive. It is like finding a broken-down typewriter with a used-up ribbon and expecting that replacing the ink will restore its function. Acetylcholine is clearly just part of the story, though an important one because it helped move the field of neuroscience from a small, esoteric collection of clinicians to the forefront of medical research. Another part of the story would emerge from research in the field of genetics.

The Genetic Story

For a long time, scientists suspected that Alzheimer's disease was genetic, or at least that there might be a genetic predisposition to its development. Some diseases are inherited with "variable penetrance," meaning that although the gene is present, only in certain cases will it actually be "expressed"—turned on by an unknown external factor. Sorting out the genetics of Alzheimer's disease proved to be very tricky. It is relatively easy to identify a genetic pattern of inheritance in a *rare* condition. In a disease that develops in nearly 50 percent of individuals over eighty-five, everyone who is afflicted will also have affected relatives, but that does not imply a genetic basis for the disease. Moreover, since Alzheimer's disease commonly has its age of onset in the eighties, and average life expectancy in America is seventy-seven for women and seventy-four for men, many people who might have been susceptible to developing Alzheimer's disease will have died before they had a chance to show signs of the disease. And given that until recently, people with dementia were commonly misdiagnosed as having other conditions altogether, such as psychosis or atherosclerosis, identifying families with a strong history of dementia was problematic.

A very small number of large families who kept careful records and tended to develop Alzheimer's disease at an unusually young age did come to medical attention. Painstaking research, often involving travel to distant parts of the globe, established the existence of a variant of Alzheimer's that was an autosomal dominant disorder: the child of an affected individual had a 50 percent chance of also getting the disease.[13] This sort of mapping of family trees disclosed that in some families the age of onset was invariably below fifty, while in others the age of onset was between fifty and sixty.

The other clue leading scientists to suspect a role for genetics was the increased prevalence of dementia in Down's syndrome. People with Down's, a genetic disorder in which there is an extra copy of chromosome 21, tend to die in their thirties and forties, too young for conventional "senile dementia." Yet when physicians looked carefully, they found that a disproportionate number of individuals with Down's showed signs of dementia by their fourth decade. Establishing that this was truly dementia took careful neuropsychological testing, since the subjects already manifested significant cognitive impairment—and were often institutionalized and did not always receive thorough medical evaluation. When autopsy specimens of people with Down's syndrome showed plaques and neurofibrillary tangles—in precisely those individuals who had evidence of dementia in life—the conclusion that Down's might provide the key to Alzheimer's disease was inescapable.

Excitement soared when the amyloid precursor protein gene was linked to chromosome 21, the very chromosome involved in Down's syndrome.[14] Within one month, four different groups confirmed the connection to chromosome 21. The prospect of a unifying theory of Alzheimer's disease was tantalizing: first a genetic defect causes the formation of a defective protein (amyloid); next, that protein is deposited in select portions of the cortex; and finally, the deposits destroy neurons, producing the clinical symptoms of Alzheimer's. But the story proved to be far more complex. Genealogically oriented researchers located a number of kindreds, large family groupings who clearly carried a genetic form of Alzheimer's disease—one that equally clearly was *not* linked to chromosome 21.[15] In fact, only 2 to 3 percent of cases of familial Alzheimer's disease were ultimately associated with the mutation on chromosome 21 (called AD1). Nonetheless, the race to actually *find* the Alzheimer's gene on chromosome 21 continued. In 1991, the DNA sequence of the mutant gene was definitively determined. Remarkably, the abnormal gene differed from the normal gene by a mutation at a single codon, or base pair in the DNA alphabet.[16] The next leg of the race entailed the search for genes responsible for the majority of cases of familial Alzheimer's.

A year later, genetics made the news again: chromosome 14 was also shown to contain a gene for Alzheimer's disease.[17] Once again, the first results were statistical: individuals in families with Alzheimer's disease who had the condition tended to have in common a "marker," a protein that was on chromosome 14, while those people in the same families without the disease did not have the same marker. Only in 1995 was the actual gene found and the amino acid sequence of its protein product determined.[18] Mutations in this gene (called AD3) currently appear to account for 70 to 80 percent of cases of familial Alzheimer's disease. The gene responsible for the remaining 20 percent of early-onset familial Alzheimer's disease remained unknown. Then, in 1995, it was hunted down on chromosome 21.[19]

In no area of Alzheimer's research has the competition been more intense than in the race to find genes responsible for the disorder. Four different groups localized a gene for familial Alzheimer's to chromosome 21 in 1987. Once again, four labs competed to identify the gene previously determined to lie somewhere along chromosome 14. A reporter for the magazine *Science* commented that "like athletes unwilling to accept defeat, a week before the *Nature* paper's publication, several of the runners-up were still springing toward the finish line."[20] The victors were euphoric, because "to people in the field, it's been a kind of a Holy Grail. . . . We've been chasing it for ten years."[21] The losers in the competition were intensely disappointed that they had, in their view, lost the opportunity to "take a trip to Stockholm," jargon for winning the Nobel Prize.

Pinning down the genetic basis of familial Alzheimer's disease is scientifically exhilarating. But understanding the pathogenesis of this form of the disease may not lead to a cure in the near future, much as the genetics and pathophysiology of diseases such as sickle cell anemia have been understood for decades, with no prospect for cure in sight. Moreover, it is far from clear that molecular studies of familial Alzheimer's disease, which accounts for 10 to 15 percent of all cases of the disease, will provide the answer to late-onset, sporadic Alzheimer's disease, which accounts for the remaining 85 to 90 percent.

A Genetic Risk Factor?

Though garden-variety, late-onset Alzheimer's disease is not attributable to a single mutation that invariably leads to disease, it may nonetheless have a genetic "risk factor." Risk factors exist for a number of today's major noninfectious killers. Heart disease is the prime example, with high blood pressure and high cholesterol and cigarette smoking the three principal risk factors. A risk factor works by increasing the probability of developing a disease, so that a person with one factor slightly increases her risk, a person with two factors further increases her risk, and a person with three risk factors faces an even greater chance of becoming ill.[22] Unlike a true "cause" of a disease, which *must* be present for the disease to develop, a risk factor may be lacking even though the disease in question is present. Not only can individuals get sick without having any "risk factors"; they can also have risk factors and escape illness. The utility of risk factor identification is in decreasing the chance of become sick by deliberately modifying risk factors: the risk of heart disease, for example, can be lowered by treating high blood pressure, by using medications or diet to lower cholesterol, and by abandoning cigarette smoking. From a public health perspective, we can have a marked effect on the incidence of disease through this approach. The effort can be dramatically effective, as with heart disease, where mortality decreased 54 percent between

1968 and 1988, only a small part of which was due to innovations such as coronary care units and coronary artery bypass surgery.[23]

One of the risk factors for coronary disease that has long been at the center of controversy is cholesterol. The "diet heart" hypothesis has had its ups and downs over the years, but it is now well established that elevated total cholesterol increases the risk of a heart attack. In the course of studying the metabolism and the genetics of cholesterol, scientists further classified cholesterol in terms of the protein molecule it traveled with in the bloodstream: those cholesterol molecules that are transported by high-density lipoprotein (HDL) turned out to have a protective effect, whereas those carried by a different protein, the low-density lipoprotein (LDL), were an even better predictor than total cholesterol of heart attack risk. As the focus of investigation shifted to the genes that regulate cholesterol handling, a new player emerged in the cholesterol field: a gene that controlled the proteins involved in cholesterol transport. Three different versions, or alleles, of this gene were found in the population, each associated with a different degree of efficiency in the handling of cholesterol. The gene was called apolipoprotein E (*APOE*), and the three alleles were designated apolipoprotein epsilon (ε) 2, 3, and 4. Studies of apolipoprotein in different populations proliferated. Quite unexpectedly, one study seemed to find a relationship between the ε4 allele and typical Alzheimer's disease.

It all started when Warren Strittmatter and Guy Salvesen, working in Allen Roses's lab at Duke University, set out to find new proteins involved in Alzheimer's. They added amyloid to cerebrospinal fluid, the fluid bathing the brain that can be sampled with a spinal tap, to see whether any proteins were attracted to the amyloid. To their surprise, they found tight binding to apolipoprotein E.[24] The discovery instantly "electrified the Alzheimer's research community" and sent biotechnology firms rushing to visit Duke. Over the next year, the Duke group worked feverishly to study the significance of this finding. Epidemiologic studies of families with a strong history of late-onset disease showed that those individuals with two copies of the *APOE*-ε4 form of the gene have eight times the risk of developing the disease as those with two

APOE-ε3 genes. Those with two copies of the rare apoE2 form have a lower than average risk. Other researchers at Duke concluded that the *APOE* gene was responsible for 75 percent of late-onset Alzheimer's.

Biochemical studies, also done at Duke, provided a theory for how apoE works. In healthy brains, the apoE3 protein (coded for by the *APOE-ε3* gene) forms a complex with another protein—which proved to be none other than tau. ApoE3 enables tau to attach to microtubules, permitting them to work properly. The alternate form—apoE4—does not bind to tau, resulting in the weakening of microtubules, and parenthetically leading to the clumping of tau into tangles. Critics of the research claim that their conclusions are suspect on methodological grounds. Roses and his group do not have an animal model: all their work is done in culture dishes and test tubes. Their results, some argue, are attributable to the massive quantities of tau and apoE used in their experiments, doses as unwarranted as their enormous conviction about the importance of their results. Competitor Rudolph Tanzi has been quoted as saying, "The jury is out as to whether apoE has any significance at all." He added, "I'm not going to undermine the importance of the discovery of *APOE* as a genetic factor, but the protein studies leave a lot to be desired," and, "It will be a while before we find the true role of apoE, if any, in the disease process."[25]

The news that apoE4 might be a risk factor for Alzheimer's disease was initially greeted with intense skepticism. After all, statistical analysis frequently demonstrates relationships that prove not to be *causal.* Sometimes statistical associations turn out to be spurious: a linkage may be found by chance alone that is not reproducible in subsequent studies. Sometimes the associations prove to be genuine, but the factor identified is a *marker* for the condition, rather than its cause. In fact, this principle underlies much of genetic research itself, since the precise location of a gene on a chromosome is often determined by virtue of its proximity to another gene that has already been identified. When the first article on a possible apoE-Alzheimer's connection appeared in 1993, the proposed linkage seemed implausible. Two years and more than two hundred articles later, apoE has become part of the Alzheimer's disease research landscape.

Much as cigarette smoking is a risk factor for heart disease, apoE4 is a risk factor for the development of nonfamilial, late-onset Alzheimer's disease. As with cigarette smoking, there are individuals with *APOE-ε4* gene (and therefore the apoE4 protein) who do not get Alzheimer's disease, and there are people with Alzheimer's disease who do not have the *APOE-ε4* allele. But unlike the cigarette smoking case, knowing that you are *APOE-ε4* positive does not give you the slightest advantage in reducing your chance of getting Alzheimer's disease. If you have the risk factor, there is absolutely nothing you can do about it.

As risk factors go, *APOE-ε4* is moderately potent—the *percent* increase in the risk of Alzheimer's disease with at least one *APOE-ε4* allele is dramatic, but the *actual* risk of the disease remains modest: only 56 percent of individuals with Alzheimer's disease have one or more *APOE-ε4* alleles, compared to 24 percent of people of the same age and gender without Alzheimer's. In the population as a whole, the lifetime risk of developing Alzheimer's disease, given current life expectancy, is 15 percent; for those with at least one *APOE-ε4* allele the lifetime risk is 29 percent, and for those with no *APOE-ε4* alleles, the risk is 9 percent.[26]

The discovery of a risk factor for Alzheimer's disease has generated tremendous concern that the test will be misused, whether in diagnosis or prediction. The availability of "presymptomatic testing" raises the specter of coerced testing and of discrimination by insurance companies based on positive results. Such testing could also lead to depression and suicide in people with positive tests and "survivor guilt" in individuals with negative tests.[27] A variety of professional organizations are meeting to develop position papers on how *APOE* testing should—or should not—be used. The consensus is that *APOE* should not routinely be used for either screening or diagnosis, that physicians and the public need to be alerted to the perils of its use, and that simple algorithms should be devised to help clinicians interpret test results that have already been obtained.[28]

The complete story of the role of apolipoproteins in Alzheimer's disease is not in yet. Linkages with amyloid as well as with tau are just now coming to light. Patients with Alzheimer's disease who have the *APOE-ε4* gene have more amyloid plaque at autopsy than those with other *APOE* variants. Research suggests that apoE proteins play a role in the clearance of amyloid—that is, the "good" apoproteins help mop up the amyloid, whereas the "bad" apoproteins are less effective in "garbage disposal." Apolipoproteins fit into the genetic studies of Alzheimer's disease as well, since the different forms of apoE are, like all proteins, determined by the genes that spell out their structure. The *APOE* genes are on chromosome 19, implicating this chromosome, along with numbers 1, 14, and 21, in the development of Alzheimer's. Ultimately, for the role of apolipoprotein E to be fully understood, its connections to both amyloid and tau will need to be clarified. For now, its significance is primarily statistical, as a factor increasing the likelihood of developing Alzheimer's.

Miscellaneous Threads

In his classic work on the growth of scientific theories, the historian of science Thomas Kuhn wrote: "In the absence of a paradigm . . . any facts that could possibly pertain to the development of a given science are likely to seem equally relevant. As a result, early fact-gathering is a far more nearly random activity."[29] Alzheimer's disease research, while far more advanced than it was ten or even five years ago, is still an immature science. There is no single, uniformly agreed upon paradigm that explains the cause and development of the disease. Not only are there rival schools—the proponents of tau (TAUists) and the adherents of amyloid (BAPtists, for beta-amyloid protein)—but there are other totally independent theories as well.

One theory that achieved wide public notice is the alleged aluminum connection. As long ago as 1897, scientists observed that aluminum injections caused degeneration of neurons in rabbits. Autopsy studies in the 1970s appeared to demonstrate higher than normal levels of aluminum in the brains of individuals diagnosed with Alzheimer's disease. This led to the hypothesis that aluminum in drinking water, or aluminum-based pots and pans, or perhaps aluminum compounds in deodorants were responsible for the development of Alzheimer's. Alzheimer's research went off on an aluminum tangent, as scientists sought to validate, reject, or elucidate the aluminum hypothesis. From an unrelated field of medicine came suggestive supporting evidence: patients with severe kidney disease requiring dialysis tended to be unable to excrete aluminum, and it accumulated in the brain. Those individuals with higher concentrations of aluminum seemed to suffer from mental deterioration that was akin to the cognitive decline in Alzheimer's disease. Epidemiologic studies looking at the aluminum exposure (through the use of antiperspirants and antacids) of patients with Alzheimer's compared to controls without the disorder found a slight, but statistically significant, difference between the two groups. Studies of the water supply in England demonstrated that the rate of Alzheimer's was very slightly higher in those districts with an aluminum concentration above a threshold level. Overall, the data, while tantalizing, suggested that aluminum might have some sort of poorly defined role but could not *account for* Alzheimer's.[30]

Another avenue of exploration that has generated a good deal of drug company interest is the nonsteroidal antiinflammatory drugs: agents such as ibuprofen (Advil or Motrin) and naproxen (Naprosyn or Aleve). In one of those wonderful serendipitous observations that are sometimes the starting point of a great discovery, physicians noticed that patients with rheumatoid arthritis, who typically use large quantities of anti-inflammatory medication, had less than the expected prevalence of Alzheimer's disease.[31] An epidemiologic study showed that in identical twins, one of whom had Alzheimer's and one of whom did not, the nonaffected twin was more likely to be a user of anti-inflammatory medication. This finding led to the speculation that Alzheimer's might be an inflammatory condition and hence treatment with antiinflammatory medication would be expected to be effective. When pathologists reanalyzed plaques and tangles microscopically, they noted all sorts of constituents that had previously been ignored. Plaques, for instance, contain inflammationfighting cells—not the same kind of cells that are typically found in an acute bacterial infection, but another variety, cells known as microglia and astrocytes, that are found exclusively in the central nervous system. Preliminary trials suggest that nonsteroidal medications may be clinically useful for

Alzheimer's.[32] Given that these same medications have a propensity to produce gastrointestinal bleeding and may cause impairment of kidney function as well as the acute, reversible form of confusion known as delirium, they will have to produce strikingly positive results for Alzheimer's to warrant their routine use.

Yet another line of investigation is the use of estrogen. Doctors have long employed estrogen replacement in postmenopausal women to avoid hot flashes and night sweats. More recently estrogen has proved to have an important role in preventing osteoporosis, the thinning of the bones that predisposes the elderly to fractures. But as the list of beneficial effects of estrogen grows, the list of possibly deleterious effects has grown as well. Estrogen clearly increases the risk of uterine cancer (in a woman who still has a uterus) and possibly increases the risk of breast cancer (though this is controversial). In the course of studying just what estrogen does and does not do biologically, estrogen receptors were found in the brain. Like other hormones, which act as modulators of important chemical reactions in the body, estrogen turns out to play a role in the brain. It even has an effect on learning and memory. The casual observation that postmenopausal women commented that their memories improved with estrogen replacement led to more systematic study. Psychological testing of women with and without estrogen confirmed slight differences. Moreover, epidemiological studies found that patients who happened to be on estrogen had a lower risk of developing Alzheimer's, though this does not mean that taking estrogen explicitly to avoid Alzheimer's will be effective, or that estrogen can be used as a treatment for Alzheimer's.[33] Currently, a large, multicenter trial is under way to answer more definitively the question of whether estrogen can help the cognitively impaired.

A final theory being extensively investigated is that toxic molecules known as free radicals play a role in causing Alzheimer's disease. The idea is that even if beta-amyloid proves to be the true culprit in Alzheimer's, we still need to understand how the amyloid accumulation destroys neurons. Stimulation of inflammatory cells (microglia and astrocytes), which then produce various harmful chemicals, is one possibility. Another is that the abnormal amyloid permits the accumulation of free radicals—that is, it prevents their normal capture and destruction before they can cause any damage. Based on this model, scientists have tested the possibility that giving anti-oxidant medications such as selegeline and vitamin E may be therapeutic in Alzheimer's disease. The one major study on the subject to date suggests that each of these drugs may be beneficial in preventing death or decline from Alzheimer's disease, although the validity of this conclusion is highly controversial.[34]

Aluminum, inflammation, estrogen deficiency, and free radicals may all play parts in Alzheimer's disease. The parts are probably relatively minor, for if any of these factors were actually the primary cause of Alzheimer's, it would not be so very difficult to ascertain whether they were even associated with the disorder. Moreover, the parts they play may be secondary rather than primary—aluminum deposits, to the extent that they occur, may be the product rather than the cause of brain damage; similarly, inflammation may be a response to rather than a precipitant of the accumulation of tau or amyloid; finally, estrogen might turn out to have a mild, nonspecific effect on improving memory but be unrelated to the basic pathology of Alzheimer's. Drug companies will no doubt try to capitalize on the reports about estrogen and anti-inflammatory medications, in the hope of expanding the market for existing medications. While these approaches could conceivably help to a very modest extent, they are extremely unlikely to make a dramatic difference in the cognitive or behavioral symptoms of Alzheimer's. Their very existence is of interest primarily as proof of how far we still have to go in understanding dementia, and of how incomplete the theoretical underpinnings of Alzheimer's research currently are.

The Whole Story

The battle rages on. Clearly, a complete explanation of Alzheimer's disease—an understanding of its cause, the mechanics of its development, and how it produces symptoms in people—will require linking *all* the components of the story. An adequate description will need to address how an alteration of one letter in one word of the genetic sentence that gives the instructions for how to make a single protein can result in Alzheimer's disease in certain families. It will need to demonstrate why plaques (with their amyloid center) and neurofibrillary tangles (with their tau core) build up in just those parts of the brain where the cholinergic neurons are concentrated. It will have to reveal how amyloid and tau interfere with neuronal functioning. And it will have to show either that exactly the same process can result from a variety of other mutations in the DNA, from high concentrations of apoE4, and from other as yet undefined abnormalities, or that the same end result can be achieved through several distinct pathways.

Just as scientists seem to be drawing together the disparate strands of Alzheimer's research, new observations are coming to light that may radically alter our understanding of the disease. Atherosclerosis, long discounted as a cause of dementia, is now recognized both as the cause of a subtype of dementia (multi-infarct dementia) and, even more surprising, as a modulating factor in Alzheimer's disease: patients with pathologic signs of Alzheimer's turn out to be far more demented if they have strokes as well.[35] Plaques and tangles, believed to be the defining characteristics of Alzheimer's disease, have recently been joined by a third, previously unrecognized brain lesion. Just as Alois Alzheimer identified neurofibrillary tangles using a special staining technique, researchers today found the new plaquelike lesions with an innovative labeling technique.[36]

If and when we have a compelling, unified conception of Alzheimer's disease, we will in all likelihood still be far away from either cure or prevention of the disorder. To date, no chronic degenerative disease can be cured. Diabetes can be treated with insulin replacement, but diabetics still suffer from problems with their heart, kidneys, and eyes because of imperfections of insulin regulation, not to mention symptoms from dramatic swings in their blood sugar levels. Congestive heart failure, in which the heart does not pump properly and fluid backs up into the lungs, can be treated with assorted medications including digoxin, diuretics, and the newer angiotensin converting enzyme (ACE) inhibitors, but the heart cannot be restored to normal functioning (except, some would argue, by heart transplantation). Renal failure, in which the kidneys can no longer filter out waste products from the bloodstream, can be effectively treated with dialysis. This approach substitutes a mechanical waste-removal system for the ailing organs but does nothing to restore the kidneys to health. And since the artificial system is neither as efficient nor as thorough as the natural one, patients on chronic dialysis eventually deteriorate despite their thrice-weekly purging of wastes.

If chronic degenerative diseases in general have been refractory to cure, chronic *neurologic* degenerative diseases have been particularly difficult to tackle. Sinemet is used to treat Parkinson's disease, a progressive disorder characterized by stiffness, slowness, and tremor, which, incidentally, is associated with its own variety of dementia in about one third of cases. Sinemet and other medications that likewise augment levels of the deficient brain chemical dopamine are tremendously beneficial drugs that can help maintain function for years, but the disease inexorably worsens. Patients with Parkinson's disease suffer a relentless downhill course, going from mild rigidity to total helplessness in a period of years. Another neurologic disease, amyotrophic lateral sclerosis or Lou Gehrig's disease, causes gradual muscle weakness until ultimately the victim cannot walk, cannot speak, cannot swallow, and finally can no longer breathe. Recently the pharmaceutical industry announced a "breakthrough" in treating this debilitating disease. According to drug company advertisements, Rilutek "protects neurons from degeneration and death" and "extends tracheostomy-free survival" (that is, survival without the need for a respirator). The small print reveals, however, that the *median* increase in survival is sixty to ninety days.

The newest and most exciting mode of attack for a variety of chronic neurologic disorders is "neuroprotective therapy," agents like Rilutek that protect neurons from all sorts of toxic substances in their environment. One kind of nerve protector, nerve growth factor (NGF), was first identified in the 1950s, and its discoverers won a Nobel prize for their work. Initially it was thought to have an effect only on the peripheral nervous system—the nerves from the spinal cord to the limbs, for example, but not on the brain itself. Then in 1986,

Franz Hefti and others found that NGF could protect cholinergic neurons, the very neurons that are among the hardest hit in Alzheimer's disease. The National Institute on Aging convened a special meeting in 1988 to decide whether to support a clinical trial of nerve growth factor in patients with Alzheimer's. They gave the project a green light, following which two biotechnology companies cloned the NGF gene and started trials of the substance to slow the advance of Alzheimer's disease.[37] Most recently, however, there have been reports of NGF's *accelerating* Alzheimer's disease. The claim that "scientists may be on the verge of beginning a new era in the treatment of degenerative brain diseases" and that neuroprotective therapy is "one of the hottest areas in neuroscience today"[38] may be more hype than truth: researchers at the University of California in Irvine found that the cholinergic nerves in Alzheimer's patients exhibit abnormal sprouting of new nerve fibers, perhaps in an attempt to compensate for lost neurons. These fibers, instead of replacing the lost neurons, seem to contribute to the formation of plaques. NGF may stimulate even more abnormal sprouting. Moreover, NGF appears to stimulate the gene coding for amyloid precursor protein, leading to increased amyloid production and still more plaques. Even if the obstacles to successful delivery of NGF to the brain can be overcome—right now the only way to get NGF to its target is by direct infusion into the brain—the possibility remains that NGF might make matters worse rather than better.

The human brain is an extraordinarily complex organ. The reductionist approach to medical problem solving, in which organic function is broken down into small, discrete component parts and organic dysfunction is attributed to failure at a single, unique point, might not be adequate to explain neurologic disorders. Brain failure may turn out to be multifactorial—to result from a combination of many separate malfunctions. But even if a single "answer" to the problem of typical Alzheimer's disease is found, prevention and treatment will most likely be far from straightforward.[39] In the event that all cases of late-onset Alzheimer's disease turn out to have a single cause, that cause will probably not yield to simple fixes. Alzheimer's disease is likely to be with us for many years to come.

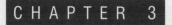

CHAPTER 3

Twilight

A telephone message awaited me when I returned from visiting my nursing home patients. The call was from Cynthia Truman, Sylvia Truman's daughter-in-law. There was a work phone number to dial—and a notation that if she was in a meeting, I was to instruct her secretary to interrupt her. My receptionist had written down "Mom acting crazy" and then "Please call" underlined three times.

I pulled Mrs. Truman's file—my office medical record—before returning the call. I had last seen her four months ago, when her son had brought her in to learn the test results. I had sent a letter to her primary care physician summarizing my findings, indicating that the most probable diagnosis was Alzheimer's disease.

Cynthia's secretary sounded relieved to hear from me. "Oh, yes, she's been waiting for your call." Moments later, I heard Cynthia's high-pitched voice. I recalled that she had seemed nervous when I had first met her; now she was frantic. "I had Mom at our house this weekend. She got up at two in the morning and left the house in her nightgown. My neighbor George just happened to see her—he's got a prostate problem or something and gets up several times during the night to go to the bathroom. He heard a noise outside and for some reason went out to check—I can't imagine why he went out in the middle of the night in his pajamas. I suppose it might have been quite a sight: two people in their eighties out on the garden path under a full moon. He was really great, my neighbor. At first Mom wouldn't come inside his house. She wouldn't come back to my house either, as she insisted she had an appointment to go to. George tried to reason with her, saying he thought her appointment probably wasn't for a few hours and she might want to put on a dress and proper shoes before going. Finally he just changed the subject and offered her a cup of tea, and she trotted in with him as though they had had a prearranged date all along. Thank goodness George knew who she was, and once he got her in the kitchen he called me." Cynthia took a deep breath. I asked whether her mother-in-law had been all right since then. "Yes and no. She hasn't wandered outside in the middle of the night. But she's been very hostile and suspicious, accusing everyone of taking her things. I didn't dare let her go back to her house all by herself. What if she went out at two A.M. again? So she's staying at our place. I hired a babysitter today—I couldn't just take off from work. I had a meeting I had to go to. I wanted to leave her with Marcia, but she's never around." She sounded apologetic, desperate, and angry at the same time.

I was about to ask whether she had called Sylvia's primary care physician. I was a consultant on this case and did not wish to overstep my bounds. "I tried reaching Dr. Boyd. He's on vacation. The covering doctor doesn't know Mom at all. And from what I've heard, he doesn't especially like dealing with older people. Nor with psychiatric sorts of things." She was imploring now. I glanced at my appointment calendar. I had a cancellation at four and I knew I could probably alleviate a great deal more pain and suffering by seeing this distressed family than by many of my other ministrations. I told Sylvia that odds were that the paranoia and confusion her mother-in-law was manifesting were part and parcel of her dementia. But since the behavior constituted an acute change, she should be checked for a new medical problem that might have triggered her symptoms. I offered the four o'clock slot. Cynthia verbally embraced me.

When Sylvia Truman came into the office later that day, she appeared different from my memory of her. On the prior encounters she had seemed a little lost. When she had looked at me head-on, her limpid doe eyes reminded me of a cornered animal's. Then, when she relaxed, thanks to a joke or a pat on the arm, hundreds of tiny wrinkles appeared in the interstices of her face: around the corners of her eyes and her mouth, even next to her nose. The mask was shattered, and the spirit underneath emerged. I had had a glimpse of the feisty matriarch she had been—proud, controlling, orderly.

Superficially, Sylvia was the same today: her hair was freshly washed and set—her daughter-in-law had seen to that—and she had had her nails done in blood red. She wore a soft beige sweater with a dark brown skirt, the pleats pressed neatly. But her eyes darted about the room, leaping from me to my desk to the certificates on the wall and back to a spot in the corner that seemed empty to me, but to which her gaze kept returning. In the brief moments of contact she looked hostile and suspicious rather than scared, as she had before. Her lids were ever so slightly closed, her shoulders were hunched forward, her legs were tightly crossed. I asked her how she was feeling.

"Fine," she barked.

I asked her if she knew why she was here.

"Cynthia." She nodded in her daughter-in-law's direction. "Cynthia thinks I'm sick."

"Cynthia's concerned about you. You weren't acting like your usual good-natured self, so she became anxious. Do you feel sick?"

"I'm fine."

I tried the laundry list approach: any headaches? sore throat? cough? diarrhea? pain when you go to the bathroom? She shook her head. "There's nothing wrong with me. And I'd like to go home now. To *my* home. She's taken me to her house and made me a prisoner. She had a security guard in the house to make sure I didn't leave."

"That was Alice," Cynthia interrupted. "Alice is practically a member of the family. She looked after my children when they were small. I asked her to come over to watch"—she stumbled a little—"to keep you company. I didn't think it was a good idea for you to be by yourself all day. I would certainly get lonely if it were me. And I just had to go to work this morning."

"That woman's a guard. You should never have let her near the children. What do you know about her past? What did she do during the war? Did you check her record? They have child molesters working in day care centers. You can't be too careful." Clearly Sylvia had been reading the newspapers or watching the news, and the more sordid stories of child abuse had made a formidable impression on her. As for the reference to the war, I was not sure to which war she was referring. The Vietnam War? The Korean War? The Second World War? The First World War? I had heard enough to conclude that not only was Sylvia confused about time—that was nothing new—but she was also paranoid.

I tried to defuse her mounting agitation. "You're right. People do have to be cautious these days. But it's Cynthia's job to worry about her children. You worried about your children when they were young—and did an excellent job bringing them up, I can see by the results. Now let's humor Cynthia by checking you over. It will just take a few minutes." Sylvia cast an angry glance at her disconsolate daughter-in-law, stood up without further hesitation, and marched after me into the examining room.

The exam, as I suspected, showed nothing. To be thorough, I sent Sylvia to the lab for another round of blood tests, but not without first handing her daughter-in-law a prescription for a low dose of Haldol, an antipsychotic medication.

"I need to be as sure as I can that there's nothing else going on," I explained to Sylvia. "But you're not on any medications that are likely to disturb your metabolism or that can build up to dangerously high levels in your blood. You're probably correct that there's nothing wrong. But being cooped up with Alice in your son's house has gotten your nerves on edge." That was, strictly speaking, true, though the gloss I chose to put on the story clearly ignored the deeper reality— that Sylvia had been taken into her son and daughter-in-law's custody because she had entered a phase of her dementia in which she tended to become paranoid.

Not everyone with dementia develops paranoia. The best estimates are that close to half do. Traditionally, hallucinations and delusions have been associated with fairly advanced dementia, but for some individuals, paranoia is the first symptom of their illness. Once paranoia develops it does not necessarily remain a permanent feature of the disease: many people go through a phase that may last for months or years, only to enter a new period in which they are calmer, less suspicious, more accepting of others.[1]

These symptoms—seeing things that aren't there, or hearing voices, or worrying about conspiracies—are identical to the symptoms that develop with psychosis, a psychiatric disturbance commonly found in schizophrenics and occasionally accompanying severe depression. But while the hallucinations of schizophrenics are usually treatable with medication (using neuroleptics, formerly referred to as major tranquilizers and sometimes called antipsychotics), the hallucinations of dementia are less responsive to treatment. Demented patients with psychotic symptoms are treated with the same drugs as schizophrenics but respond less reliably.[2]

Nursing home advocacy groups and others have strongly criticized the use of antipsychotic medications for patients with dementia, particularly in the nursing home setting: patients have been found to be excessively sedated, to be suffering from side effects of medications, or to be maintained on medicines despite their lack of efficacy. Certainly the antipsychotic medications can produce lethargy, though different members of the neuroleptic family produce different side effects: some, such as chlorpromazine (Thorazine), have a great propensity for sedation, and others, such as haloperidol (Haldol), have a much smaller chance of causing sedation. Patients, particularly those who are elderly, are variable in their susceptibility to sedation, so some people will become sleepy even on the seldom soporific haloperidol, while some will remain alert and vigilant even on drugs such as thioridazine (Mellaril), which are far more commonly sedating. Sedation is not the only potential side effect of the neuroleptics. Because they block the neurotransmitter dopamine, they can produce a picture very much like Parkinson's disease, complete with stiffness, tremor, and a shuffling gait. Again, the neuroleptics can be arranged along a spectrum, with some drugs far more likely than others to affect movement. Unfortunately, the medicines that are the least sedating are the ones most likely to cause parkinsonism, and, conversely, those that are least likely to cause parkinsonism are the most likely to cause lethargy; there is no one medication that is devoid of the risk of adverse effects. The sedating forms are also apt to cause low blood pressure, which in turn increases the risk of falling and may also worsen confusion.

The neuroleptics have also gotten a bad rap because the caregivers who administer them in some nursing homes have been found to be abysmally ignorant of their side effects. They continue to give patients these medications even if the patients become sleepy or fall or have a tremor, because the caregivers are unaware that such symptoms might connote medication toxicity and warrant follow-up by a physician. As a result of publicity about the misuse of antipsychotics in residents of nursing homes, a federal law was passed mandating clear documentation of the indications for use of these drugs, careful monitoring for side effects, and periodic discontinuation of the medications. Studies conducted in nursing homes after the introduction of the new law demonstrated a marked reduction in the prescribing of antipsychotic drugs, without any measurable adverse effect on patients.[3]

For all the concern about the potential undesirable effects of antipsychotics, they have a legitimate role in the management of patients with dementia. At least one third of the time the medicine works, and if one particular variety of antipsychotic must be discontinued due to intolerable side effects, often its cousin can be successfully substituted. The reality is that paranoid delusions—such as Sylvia Truman's erroneous conviction that Alice, a trusted family friend, was out to get her—are not merely unpleasant for family and caregivers; they are frightening to the patient herself. While there is little justification for the use of strong medicine for the purpose of preventing patients from calling out incessantly, a behavior that is noxious to third parties but unobjectionable from the point of view of the perpetrator, there is ample reason to seek to obliterate alarming hallucinations and delusions.

A few days later I received a message that Sylvia had improved and was determined to go home. Cynthia brought her mother-in-law to the office for me to check for side effects of the medication and to help decide whether Sylvia should live home alone.

Sylvia was more animated than when I had last seen her before. She was a little testy—she failed to see why anyone else should have a voice in planning her life. "I'm fine," she insisted. "I think I had a virus yesterday." She meant when she had come in the previous week. "I like visiting John and Cynthia. But they both work during the day. And when the children come home, the house is awfully noisy. I can't hear myself think. It's okay to come up on the weekends, but I'm much more comfortable in my own house."

She was right: being in an alien environment was itself disorienting. She had lived in her home for nearly fifty years and knew where the light switches were, where she kept her things, where to find the telephones. Now that she was sleeping through the night again, she was probably reasonably safe on her own from evening on. But what of daylight hours, when she might be tempted to turn on the stove to make a cup of tea, or go out by herself? Spring had come to New England: the crocuses were in bloom, the leaves were just turning green, and the park near Sylvia's house was filled with chirping birds and gleeful children delighted to be able to play outdoors at last. But the children had parents or baby-sitters to accompany them; Sylvia did not. Would she find her way home? Would she remember to watch for oncoming traffic when she stepped into the street? Would her hunger and thirst mechanism be adequate to remind her to go home for lunch?

I delayed addressing the safety questions while I examined Sylvia for evidence of parkinsonism. She was not stiff; she had no tremor. Her walking was brisk, without the hesitation or small steps characteristic of Haldol toxicity. Her blood pressure was excellent and remained normal when she moved from sitting to standing. She did not appear listless or lethargic, and Cynthia reported that she was appropriately alert during the day and slept well at night. So far, the Haldol had caused no problems. Sylvia was still quick to jump to the conclusion that her bag had been stolen whenever she misplaced it, but she readily conceded that no one would want to take her glasses or her slippers. Once the missing items were located, she acknowledged that her memory was not what it used to be. Sylvia was not pleased to be left with Alice every day, but she no longer alluded to Alice's nefarious past or talked of child molesters. In short, she was still suspicious but not flagrantly paranoid. Her overriding desire was to return home.

I tried the direct approach: Sylvia's memory wasn't so good anymore, so Cynthia and I were worried about her safety.

"I may not have a very good memory, but that doesn't mean I can't be alone," she shot at me. "You two are in cahoots," she went on. "You're up to something." Evidently she still had a tendency to see the world in a paranoid light, though the light was no longer as glaring as previously.

"We are both concerned about you," I admitted. "I'm also thinking about how lonely it must be for you." I decided there was no point in confronting Sylvia with her deficits: she clearly had no recollection of our discussion about dementia, and she would vigorously deny that there was anything significantly wrong with her cognitive function. I remembered that the strategy of making changes so as to humor her children had worked to persuade her to stop driving; I tried to capitalize on this approach. "How about if you went home—to your home—and your housekeeper came every day in the afternoon for a while to do some errands and get dinner ready and do whatever cleaning was necessary? And so you won't be lonely during the day, before the housekeeper arrives, we could arrange for you to go to a special program for senior citizens." Sylvia, who until now had been skeptical but receptive, put her foot down.

"I'm not interested in spending my time with a bunch of old people." I couldn't help smiling, just a little bit. I turned to Cynthia to prevent Sylvia from seeing my expression, and found she was suppressing a giggle.

"But, Mom, how old do you think you are?"

"I know I'm eighty-two. But I don't feel old. I don't use one of those things—what do you call it—that old people walk with—"

"A walker?"

"Yes, a walker. I don't need a cane, and I haven't been sick a day in my life. I don't want to be cooped up with people who aren't like me."

"Fair enough. But I'm not so sure the other members of the group are so different from you. I think there are lots of people who live alone and appreciate having company."

"If I want company, I'll go see my own friends," Sylvia flashed back.

"Come on, Mom. How often do you end up seeing your friends?"

"Well, I was seeing them pretty often until you made me give up driving."

My scheme seemed to be backfiring. I couldn't very well suggest that attending an adult day care program was just another change she should make to please her family, like forgoing driving, since she already felt deprived by her loss of freedom. Nor could I persuade her that spending six hours a day in a supervised setting with a nurse to monitor blood pressure and administer medications and with organized activities was just the thing for her. She did not see herself as old or needing supervision or incapable of finding companionship on her own.

"How about this," I suggested, ignoring the comment about driving. "How about if you and Cynthia—or Marcia or John— visit the program that's very near where you live. It meets in the Presbyterian church in your neighborhood. Then decide, once you've seen for yourself."

Sylvia scowled. "They probably do arts and crafts or play bingo. I hate bingo and I stopped doing arts and crafts when I was six." She was unfortunately right that many programs for the elderly infantilize their clientele: they transplant curricular materials from nursery school to the senior center. But some programs also include discussion groups, "adopt a grandparent" sessions in which older people are paired with a child, and, at the request of the participants, sophisticated card games such as bridge.

"I don't know exactly what goes on at the center in your community. That's why it would make sense for you to visit."

Sylvia and Cynthia got up to leave. Clearly, considerable family pressure would be necessary for day care to work out. But adult day care was a way for Sylvia to remain in her own home. As part of a package that included a private housekeeper for a few hours each weekday afternoon and transportation to day care at 8 A.M. with a return trip at 2 P.M., it offered the possibility of preserving independence in the community while promoting safety and social contact.

* * *

I learned from the geriatric social worker, Nancy Kingsley, a few weeks later, that Sylvia had been enrolled in an adult day care program. Every day she threatened to refuse to go, every day she protested that she was not at all like the other people in the center—and every day she was ready when the van arrived to transport her to the center. The plan for Sylvia Truman's care was complex and therefore tenuous. Its success depended on her agreeing to go to day care, on the reliability of her housekeeper, on her remaining reasonably safe alone at night, and on her family's taking her into their homes for the weekends. If the housekeeper called in sick or day care was closed for a holiday or Sylvia's children went on vacation, there was a crisis. But these were small crises, minor perturbations against which the family could insure themselves with an array of backup plans. The Truman family was pleased that the system they had arranged was working as well as it was, but they sensed that the package could fall apart at any time.

The crisis the Trumans had been expecting arrived without warning just as John and Cynthia were preparing to go on vacation. Their suitcases were packed and they were ready to leave for the airport. They had taken Sylvia out for dinner the evening before: she had been in good spirits and had eaten an elaborate meal. They were drawing the blinds and setting the timer on the living room lamps when the phone call came. It was the driver of the day care van. Sylvia had not been outside waiting for him when he arrived. Nor had she come to the door when he rang. If John and Cynthia had a key, he suggested, they might want to zip over and check up on her.

John's mind went into overdrive. He could not call his sister—she lived forty minutes away. There was no choice but to go over himself. He would go with Cynthia and they would take their luggage. If Mom was all right—perhaps she had overslept or had been in the shower when the van had come—they would head directly to the airport from Sylvia's house. If she wasn't all right—he could not proceed with this line of thinking—they would do whatever had to be done.

When John and his wife arrived, the house was quiet. Sylvia sometimes listened to the radio or turned on the television to keep her company, which might make it difficult for her to hear the doorbell. There were no lights on, at least none visible from the front of the house, but it was a sunny morning, and Sylvia's kitchen and living room, where she spent most of her time, were brightly lit at this hour. Grimly and apprehensively, as he reported to me later, John pressed the buzzer. He tried once again a half minute later, and then he and Cynthia let themselves in.

"Mom? Are you here? It's John and Cynthia." Could she have gone somewhere? Could she be lost? They checked all the rooms on the first floor: she was not, as John had secretly hoped, napping on the living room sofa. She was not sipping tea in the kitchen, oblivious to the mounting anxiety she was generating. She was not in her bedroom. The bathroom door was shut. Cynthia opened it and found her mother-in-law lying on the floor. Cynthia gasped, John came running, and Sylvia woke up.

She had fallen during the night when she had gotten up to go to the bathroom. She thought she had tripped—she was not quite sure how it happened. She hit the floor with a tremendous crash, her head just missing the sink as she went down. The pain had been excruciating. She had cried and called out, but no one could hear her. Her Lifeline—the special device she was supposed to wear around her neck to call for help in an emergency—lay on the night table next to her bed. And despite multiple trials, she had been utterly unable to get up. She had lain on the bathroom floor, in severe pain, for hours. Finally, exhausted with weeping, she had fallen asleep.

John called an ambulance and minutes later she was in my hospital's emergency room. An X ray conclusively demonstrated what was suspected clinically: Sylvia had broken her hip. She was given an injection of Demerol for pain and transferred to a hospital bed. Surgery was scheduled for the same afternoon.

The Trumans spent their vacation at the hospital instead of in the Bahamas. When I saw John at his mother's bedside, a day after the operation, he joked that it had been a great way to free up his calendar so he'd have plenty of time to visit his mother in the hospital. He added that it was the last time he would purchase nonrefundable tickets for anything. I commiserated with him and then started my evalua-

tion of his mother, whom I had been asked to see in consultation because she was reported to be confused and combative.

I said hello to Sylvia, introducing myself. She looked at me
blankly, registering no recognition. "Do you know where you
are?" I asked her.

"Of course I know," she snarled at me.

"And what is the name of this place?"

"It's Johnny's." Her son intervened, explaining that Johnny's
Luncheonette was a few blocks away from her house.

"I don't think so," I responded gently. "You're in the hospital. You fell at home and broke your hip."

She turned to face me, incredulous. "I did?"

"Yes. Your son found you on the floor and brought you to
the hospital. You had surgery yesterday." I showed her the
incision on her thigh.

"Well, well," Sylvia commented, closed her eyes, and went
to sleep.

I examined her briefly, looking for causes of postoperative
confusion, or delirium. She did not have a fever, her breathing was calm, and her lungs were clear, all arguing against
pneumonia. When she was awake, she did not appear to be in
pain. She was blissfully unaware of both the fall and the fracture. I reviewed her medications: in addition to the anes-
thetics used during surgery, which were gradually wearing off,
she was on a hefty dose of Demerol for pain and a strong
sleeping pill at night. I suggested to the orthopedists that
while pain control was certainly important—and pain itself
can cause confusion—Mrs. Truman did not seem to require
narcotics any longer. She might do well with plain Tylenol
administered around the clock so as to maintain constant
levels in her blood. I pointed out that Sylvia would be better
off without a sleeping potion, but that if she was truly restless
and unable to sleep at night, a medication whose effects
would not linger during daylight hours was preferable to the
long-acting medication she had received the previous night.

When I came back to see Sylvia the following day, I hoped
to find her out of bed, walking with the guidance of a physical
therapist, and back to her baseline mildly confused self. I had
the first inkling that all was not well when I heard her
shrieking halfway down the hospital corridor.

She was lying in bed, her hands tied to the bedrails with

soft restraints—padded cuffs wrapped around her wrists, with straps attached. She was wearing a "Posey" jacket—a vest fitted over her hospital johnny that was tied to the back of the bed, effectively preventing her from sitting up. She was wide awake, terror in her eyes, alternately screaming "nurse" and "mama." I untied her hands and raised the head of the mechanical bed so that she was sitting up. I sat next to her on the bed and asked her if there was something that would make her more comfortable.

I expected her to say she wanted to go home, or that she was in pain. Instead she became docile and requested a drink of water. I handed her a cup. She drank avidly, noisily.

At this juncture the nurse caring for her during the current shift came in and glared reprovingly at my handiwork. "She kept ripping out her intravenous, so she had to be restrained," the nurse explained.

"Does she really need an intravenous line?" I asked innocently. "What's she getting by vein?"

The nurse acknowledged that Sylvia did not need the catheter in her vein for medications: the few medications the doctors had prescribed were pills. "She's not taking much in the way of fluids, so she needed the intravenous for hydration."

I nodded sympathetically. Sylvia did seem mildly dehydrated. But she was thirsty now and wanted to drink. The day before she had been too lethargic to drink much; now she was eager to drink but she needed access to fluids. That meant leaving her hands untied and keeping a pitcher and cup within easy reach.

"Maybe that would be all right," the nurse allowed skeptically. "But she still needs the Posey jacket or she'll climb out of bed. It's not safe for her to walk unassisted, but she doesn't remember that. Half the time she doesn't know where she is, and she doesn't believe me when I tell her she broke her hip." This was a tough one. The Posey only exacerbated Sylvia's agitation. But until it was safe for her to get up on her own, she had to be protected from herself. On the other hand, the best strategy for improving her mobility and rendering her independent was to get her out of bed and on her feet. As long as she was confused and belligerent, the therapists were unable to work with her. She typically could not focus on the instructions they gave her, and when she did pay attention, she forgot what she had been told within minutes.

The only satisfactory way out of this difficult situation was to have someone stay with Sylvia at all times. The effect of a human presence had been striking. Sylvia's nurse agreed: as soon as she came in the room, Sylvia calmed down. But seconds after she left, the cries of "nurse" or "help" resumed. Sylvia was anxious to the point of panic. She could not remember where she was or what had happened to her; she had no idea of what would happen to her next, and she found herself inexplicably unable to move. Haldol—the medication Sylvia was already taking because of her history of paranoia—can sometimes help control the agitation. With luck, an infection or a medication may be responsible for the heightened confusion. In that case, treating the infection or discontinuing the offending medication could resolve the problem. With Sylvia, her illness or, in some undefined way, the hospitalization itself, triggered the delirium. Time is the great healer, but unfortunately, if recovery takes days, the rehabilitative process is correspondingly delayed.

It is increasingly commonplace for patients who have had hip surgery to go to a nursing home rather than to return home. With the advent of "diagnosis-related groups" (DRGs), hospitals are paid a fixed rate by Medicare for a given medical problem. There is variability depending on the geographic area in which the hospital is located, and certain complications justify an increase in the standard reimbursement. But for the most part, a patient with a hip fracture is expected to require a four- to five-day hospital stay, and the hospital will be paid only for a five-day hospitalization, even if the patient develops delirium and lingers for ten days. The hospital has a clear incentive to keep patients for the DRG-allotted time and no longer. In most hospitals, the result is that patients are discharged "quicker and sicker." They are booted out as soon as they no longer need intravenous medication or complex diagnostic tests, as soon as they are medically stable. If it is time to leave but they are unable to return home because they are still confused or too weak to care for themselves, then the choice is between a nursing home and a rehabilitation hospital. The problem is that rehabilitation hospitals have their own special admissions process: a patient's doctor cannot simply admit him to the rehabilitation facility the way he could admit him to an acute care hospital. The patient is typically screened for suitability by a representative of the rehab. Will he be able to tolerate three hours of therapy daily, the intensity mandated for the hospital to qualify for Medicare reimbursement? Is he showing sufficient progress while at the acute hospital to justify concluding that he would continue to improve in the rehab and, in a matter of weeks, be able to go home? If not, he is rejected and usually has no alternative but to enter a nursing home, or skilled nursing facility, where, if he is fortunate, he will receive physical therapy, though at a less vigorous pace.

The catch-22 is that DRGs mean hip fracture patients are branded ready for discharge in just a few days, at which time many are too weak or confused to pass the admissions test for rehabilitation. Thus a smaller percentage meet the criteria for acceptance to a rehab hospital since the introduction of DRGs than previously; they end up in nursing homes instead. And while the transfer to a nursing home is often intended to be temporary, in one third of cases it proves to be permanent.[4]

Sylvia Truman was fortunate that her family possessed the resources and the will to hire round-the-clock private duty nurses for her. While she was hospitalized, the nurses provided the soothing words and reassuring pats that worked at least as well as high-dose Haldol, without any of the side effects. Under the nurses' watchful eyes, she could be unbound, allowed out of bed, and progressively permitted to walk.

By the fifth postoperative day, Sylvia's delirium was lifting. She had not, however, adjusted to her new environment: there were too many new and alien aspects of her hospital existence to expect her to recall, let alone comprehend, all that was happening. Even the routine part of her stay was marred by flux. A hospital nurse was assigned to her, who checked her vital signs, changed her dressing, and administered her medications. But there was a new nurse every eight-hour shift, and the weekend nurses were different from the weekday nurses. Sylvia shared her room with a roommate, and her bed remained the one near the window; however, the occupant of the second bed changed three times in the course of Sylvia's weeklong stay. Her first roommate was discharged home at the height of Sylvia's agitation; her second roommate suffered a cardiac arrest and died; and her third roommate, who had incurred multiple fractures in a car accident and was wrapped in so many bandages she looked like a mummy, moved in two days before Sylvia was discharged.

Sylvia was discharged to a nearby rehabilitation hospital that believed she was lucid enough to benefit from their program. Or perhaps they were willing to give her a chance, knowing that she had sufficient resources to pay privately for nursing home care, should she do poorly in rehab and be unable to return home. Understandably, rehabilitation hospitals did not want to be saddled with patients who were "disposition problems," patients for whom Medicare would no longer pay but who could not be discharged home. Because Sylvia Truman had substantial savings, she would not have to wait long for a room in a nursing home.

The hope, of course, of both the rehab facility and Sylvia's family was that she would spend a few weeks getting intensive physical therapy and then be able to get out of bed, walk, and shower independently, as she had done previously. Ultimately, this episode in Sylvia's life had a happy ending: her walking improved and she went back home. But her stay in the rehab was perhaps even more fraught with difficulties than her stay in the hospital: at least in the hospital, Sylvia had been passive—the physicians had operated on her, they had given her medication. At the rehab, the onus for getting better was on Sylvia herself—the therapists expected her to participate actively in her treatment.

Her arrival was auspicious. It was a sunny day, and her room overlooked a small but impeccably maintained flower garden. The difficulty of being in another strange place was tempered by the attractiveness of her surroundings. She arrived in time for lunch and pronounced the food infinitely superior to the dry, overcooked fare she had come to expect at the acute care hospital. The physical therapist who evaluated her was young, sporting a ponytail and a short denim skirt, reminding Sylvia of her granddaughter. She was cheerful and good-natured and confident that Sylvia would progress beautifully. Sylvia had not gotten much encouragement in recent months and especially not in the last few days. She had come to sense that most of the people who worked with her expected her to fail. Being with this young woman who was sure she would triumph was uplifting.

The trouble began when the sun went down. Sylvia dozed off after supper and then woke up when a nurse came in to check her blood pressure. Startled, she was convinced she was at her daughter Marcia's house but did not understand why Marcia was nowhere to be seen. She became increasingly frantic, and as her anxiety mounted her delusions intensified. The nurse was transformed into a spy who had tied Marcia up in the basement. A telephone call to an exhausted but unfettered Marcia finally persuaded Sylvia that her fears were exaggerated. She remained convinced she was in Marcia's home but was distracted from her quest for Marcia by a medical drama on television.

The following day was rocky as well. Sylvia tired after twenty minutes of therapy and refused to do any more exercises. When the therapist returned a few hours later to pick up where she had left off, Sylvia had forgotten all the exercises she had been taught earlier. In the evening she "sundowned" again. This time her delusions were less vivid and correspondingly less distressing. She was given a tranquilizer, a benzodiazepine, to temper her anxiety. The drug wore off during the night, and Sylvia woke up abruptly, frightened and in pain. She knew she was in the hospital and she knew enough not to get up on her own, but she could not figure out how to summon help. She had no recollection of the "call light," suspended by a cord and clipped to the side of her bed, within easy reach. Her inhibitions were in working order so she did not dare call out. Instead, she lay in bed and cried.

The rehab hospital placed two demands on Sylvia Truman that were simply beyond her capabilities: it expected her to learn and remember totally new material (exercises that bore little resemblance to anything in her experience), and it assumed that her problem-solving ability was normal (that finding herself in a novel predicament, she could figure out how to extricate herself). While much of Sylvia's memory was still intact—her memory of facts and concepts about the world, for instance—those aspects of memory necessary for the acquisition of new habits were terribly impaired.[5] More-over, she had trouble using either logic or her knowledge of the world to cope with new and unexpected situations.[6]

After ten long and frustrating days at the rehab, the staff felt they had achieved as much as was possible with Sylvia Truman. Whether because of their expertise or despite it, Sylvia had progressed sufficiently so that she could walk without assistance on level ground. Her family agreed to set up a bedroom for her on the first floor, reinstitute day care, and hire an aide for the evening hours. With a complex and precarious mix of community services in place to keep her afloat, Sylvia Truman went back to her own home.

CHAPTER 4

Alzheimer's Disease— the History

Some days I see dementia everywhere. I notice an elderly woman on the sidewalk, dressed in a peculiar outfit, her shirt and slacks clashing, her sweater soiled, and I wonder if she's got it. I have a telephone conversation with an eighty-year-old relative who repeats herself and doesn't seem to grasp a very simple idea, and I worry that it's starting. The son of a ninety-five-year-old patient, himself about seventy, asks me exactly the same questions he asked me last week, which I happen to know are also the same questions he asked the nurse at his mother's nursing home this morning, and I ask myself whether he, too, could be developing Alzheimer's disease.

As I enter the notes in the medical records of one demented patient after another, I wonder how it could possibly be that, until twenty-five years ago, physicians believed cognitive loss was a normal part of aging. The term "Alzheimer's disease" was coined back in 1910, based on Alois Alzheimer's findings in Frau D. (see Chapter 2). But at the time, the label was applied exclusively to younger individuals. Scientists presumed that dementia was a *disease* when it occurred in those under sixty and that it was *natural* when it was found in older people. Surely it has always been obvious that while most people in their eighties develop mild forgetfulness (an apparently normal concomitant of aging), some elderly demonstrate extreme confusion (more consistent with a disease process). Or could the disease as we know it today, a disorder of epidemic proportions in the very old, be a new condition altogether? As I investigated the history of Alzheimer's disease and other forms of dementia, I discovered that conceptions of "normal" cognitive function in old age turn out to have varied considerably over the centuries. The views reflected changes both in scientific knowledge and in societal attitudes toward the elderly.

Dementia in the Remote Past

In theory, what we refer to today as dementia might be a new disease. The great plagues of the twentieth century, Ebola and Lassa fever and AIDS, do appear to be caused by relatively new viruses, or at least by viruses that only recently began attacking human beings. Dementia, however, seems to have been around as long as people have lived to be old enough to develop it. Plato (429–348 B.C.) commented that a man "in a state of madness or under the influence of old age" could not be held responsible for his crimes.[1] Plato did not attribute the poor judgment of old age to brain dysfunction: he blamed it on a weakness of the soul. Nonetheless, he clearly recognized that thinking is sometimes dramatically impaired in the aged. He acknowledged implicitly that some old people are perfectly rational; hence cognitive decline is not inevitably associated with aging.[2]

Writing two hundred fifty years after Plato, the Roman statesman Cicero (106–43 B.C.), asserted that "the senile folly called dotage is characteristic not of all old men but only of the frivolous." Cicero, in what could not have been a totally self-serving argument since he himself did not survive to old age, maintained that old men in general were wiser and more capable than younger men.[3] Evidently he did not regard impaired reasoning as a natural part of aging.

Only in the writings of Galen (A.D. 130–200), do we find an eminent physician recording for posterity his thoughts on mental function in old age. Like his nonmedical contemporaries, Galen recognized that, at least in cases of extreme debility, the elderly manifested "imbecility." Galen believed that aging was essentially a process of drying out and shriveling up: mental decline was due to "evaporation of corporeal heat and moisture."[4] Galen's views, though often based on

animal dissections and idiosyncratic, unsubstantiated theories, shaped both medical thinking in general and prejudices
about dementia in particular for over a thousand years.

The close of the Middle Ages brought no dramatic change
in the popular image of old age. The life cycle, for those
fortunate enough to survive to old age, ended with decay.
William Shakespeare (1564–1616) called old age a second
childhood—a period of both physical and mental weakness.
In his description of the seven ages of man, he had this to say
about old age:

> Last scene of all,
> What ends this strange eventful history,
> Is second childishness and mere oblivion,
> Sans teeth, sans eyes, sans taste, sans every thing.[5]

Among those who made it to adulthood, a few, throughout recorded history, lived into their sixties and seventies.
Truly old people—those over eighty—were a rarity and were
regarded with awe by virtue of their sheer existence. Despite
the wonder that colored the perception of the elderly, it
was obvious that some of the oldest old lost their minds as
they aged.

Old age was clearly not a hot topic for the millennia during which life expectancy was thirty years. At the same time,
among those who gave the matter some thought, there was a
nagging sense that not everybody lost his mind as he got old:
dementia was not normal, "imbecility" was precipitated by
"frivolity" or "weakness of the soul." But only when physicians
and the general public started thinking in terms of specific
diseases rather than isolated symptoms, and from there
moved on to recognize that a given disease had a particular
cause, did they see dementia as a *disorder*, worthy of study.

The Specificity of Disease

It is difficult for me to imagine how my predecessors saw
illness, when I so naturally think of pneumonia and AIDS
and breast cancer as discrete diseases. In previous eras, the
boundaries between diseases were blurred, minor illnesses

were thought to transform into serious ones, and emotions were seen as the catalyst that tipped the balance between health and sickness.[6] The idea of a disease as a unique entity, with characteristic symptoms resulting from observable changes in the body's tissues, is the product of the nineteenth century.[7] Once physical symptoms were grouped into disease categories, it was still a leap to make comparable groupings for mental symptoms. The first physicians to think about *mental* illness in a similar light—as a problem that must have a cause, a course, and potentially a cure—were a French triumvirate, Philippe Pinel, his student Jean Esquirol, and Esquirol's student, Jean Martin Charcot. These three men got their clinical experience working in the monstrous almshouses, the Salpêtrière and Bicêtre, which were home to the poor, the elderly, the insane, the crippled, and the orphaned of Paris. The three physicians made names for themselves trying to improve the quality of care of the five thousand or more subjects under their jurisdiction, and by elevating the asylums into premier teaching and research institutions. They each developed a reputation by devising progressively more elaborate systems of classification of pathology based on their observation of clinical symptoms.

Historians attribute the first modern usage of the term *dementia* to Pinel (1745–1826), who wrote of "*démence*," or dementia, in his *Treatise on Insanity*.[8] Pinel spoke of the "incoherence of the mental faculties" in his patients, which certainly is compatible with dementia. But when he went on to state that it was characterized by a rapid succession of unrelated ideas, I realized he was at least as likely to have meant schizophrenia, which is characterized by the haphazard stringing together of ideas, as he was to have meant the cognitive impairment that is today called dementia. Just how far Pinel's thinking was from contemporary ideas became even more apparent when I found that he believed that "dementia" originated in the stomach and that it could be triggered by disappointed ambition or unrequited love.[9]

Pinel's successor, Esquirol (1772–1840), came a little closer to the current view in his book, *Mental Maladies*. He defined dementia as "a cerebral affection, usually chronic and unattended by fever, and characterized by a weakness of the sensibility, understanding, and will. Incoherence of ideas, and a want of intellectual and moral spontaneity, are the signs of this affection." Some of his demented patients, like Pinel's, were undoubtedly schizophrenics—such as the twenty-nine-year-old and the twenty-seven-year-old about whom he wrote. But Esquirol tried to distinguish between different variants of dementia: the type afflicting young people, which he attributed to menstrual disorders, masturbation, and domestic arguments, and the type afflicting older people, which he blamed on "the progress of age." Among the 184 cases of "dementia" he reported observing at the Salpêtrière, he classified 19 percent as senile dementia. He probably correctly diagnosed some cases of dementia in his older subjects, writing that "man, passing insensibly into the vale of years, loses his sensibility, along with the free exercise of his understanding, before reaching the extreme of decrepitude. This form of mental disease is gradually established. It commences with a weakening of the memory, especially with respect to recent impressions." However, forced to rely exclusively on qualitative clinical observations to form his classification scheme, with no recourse to pathology to validate his categorization, Esquirol could not clearly demarcate schizophrenia, depression, and dementia.[10]

Brilliant as he was, Jean Martin Charcot (1825–93), the last and most distinguished of the three giants, could not get much further than Pinel and Esquirol in his understanding of dementia. He did acknowledge that dementia was a disease, and he began trying to correlate symptoms with physical changes. He observed, for instance, that dementia was typically associated with cerebral atrophy, or wasting, which was clearly visible on gross examination of the brain at autopsy. But until physicians moved from defining disease exclusively by categorizing symptoms to focusing on pathology, they would be unable to solidify the concept of dementia. Seeing disease primarily in terms of the physical changes induced in the human body was the contribution of the great German pathologist Rudolf Virchow (1821–1902). Virchow was particularly impressed by the alterations he saw in blood vessels under the microscope. He regarded atherosclerosis, the narrowing of blood vessels, as the cause of old age in general, and atherosclerosis of cerebral vessels as the cause of mental deterioration in particular.

The discovery of microbes was the critical last step that led nineteenth-century physicians to embrace the idea of the specificity of disease. Thanks to the germ theory, disease became more concrete. At least for infections, each disease had an observable etiology. Patients developed similar clusters of symptoms—fever and cough, or a red throat with enlarged tonsils, or burning and frequency of urination; the specific symptom clusters were associated with particular pathologic changes (pneumonia with pus in the lung tissue, meningitis with inflammation of the lining of the brain); and each symptom complex appeared to be caused by a unique microbiological agent. While the experience of illness varied from individual to individual, depending on the social circumstances, the personality, and the age and overall well-being of the victim, diseases themselves were invariant. Dementia was no exception.

By the time Alois Alzheimer (1864–1915) served as a physician in the mental asylum at Frankfurt, Germany, the idea of the specificity of disease was well established. It made perfectly good sense to physicians to view progressive loss of memory, disorientation, and the inability to care for oneself as a distinct disease. When Alzheimer studied the brain of Frau Auguste D., his first demented patient under sixty, and found neurofibrillary tangles, he concluded that these ghosts of old neurons were the pathologic basis for Frau D.'s dementia: "Clinically the patient presented such an unusual picture that the case could not be categorized under any of the known diseases. Anatomically the findings were different from all other known disease processes."[11]

Alzheimer did not know the cause of those changes. But his observations of new and peculiar abnormalities in the brain of a woman suffering from a syndrome of mental deterioration implied a new disease. There is nothing surprising in Alzheimer's having drawn the conclusion that all people like Mrs. D. were afflicted with the same malady. Instead of assuming that fifty-year-olds with progressive problems in memory, judgment, and language might have a dozen different conditions, he suspected that they would all prove to have the same pathology and hence the identical medical condition. What is remarkable is not that a neuropathologist in the early 1900s should see all the Mrs. D.s of the world as cut from a single cloth; what is fascinating is that he did not accept that individuals older than Mrs. D. with precisely the same symptoms and the identical clinical course were affected by the same disease.

The possibility that "presenile dementia" and "senile dementia" were the same entity did cross Alois Alzheimer's mind. While he was quite definitive in his initial report that the case of Frau D. could not be made to "fit" into any of the "known disease categories," and asserted that "we are apparently confronted with a distinctive disease process," he was less certain in a subsequent paper written four years later. He started out arguing that "since the patient was only 56 years of age . . . this case could not be categorized among known disorders." But then, referring to the work of others on plaques and tangles, he added: "the question . . . arises as to whether the cases of disease which I considered peculiar are sufficiently different clinically and histologically to be distinguished from senile dementia or whether they should be included under that rubric." He then concluded that "there is no tenable reason to consider these cases as caused by a specific disease process. *They are senile psychoses, atypical forms of senile dementia.*" (Emphasis in original.)[12] However, in 1910, Emil Kraepelin, the distinguished psychiatrist who also happened to be Alzheimer's boss, wrote in the revised edition of his textbook of psychiatry that there was a dementing illness called "Alzheimer's disease" that exclusively afflicted those under sixty.[13] With a single flourish of the pen, Kraepelin gave the newly identified disorder a name and a constituency.

A careful reading of Kraepelin's work shows that he, too, had his misgivings. In a lecture on "senile imbecility," published in 1904, several years before Alzheimer's pivotal observations, Kraepelin distinguished between mild forgetfulness in old age, which he regarded as normal, and "senile imbecility," which he was not willing to call normal, but nonetheless attributed to "the morbid changes of old age." Kraepelin delineated in crisp, clear terms the usual course, what we today refer to as the natural history, of dementia. He described a patient who, at age seventy-two, was so forgetful that she could not find her way around the house. Often she could not remember whether or not she had eaten lunch. She thought her daughter was her sister and often spoke of her long-dead parents as though she had seen them that very day. Over time, she became irritable and restless. She refused to go to bed at night and was up before dawn. Ultimately, she developed "catatonic features"—what we would regard today as the final stage of dementia. Kraepelin balked at calling this severe form of "senile imbecility" normal aging. He also balked at calling it dementia praecox—what would later be known as schizophrenia, another disease that caused catatonia. Instead, he threw up his hands and said that perhaps further developments in the field of pathological anatomy would help clarify the "clinical position" of this disorder.[14]

When Alzheimer reported brain changes that appeared to correlate with this syndrome in a fifty-five-year-old, Kraepelin reacted with caution. He wrote that the "clinical significance of Alzheimer's disease is not yet clear." Kraepelin acknowledged that the anatomic findings suggested that Alzheimer had found an "especially severe form of senile imbecility," but then, evidently rebutting his own argument, said this cannot be because the illness Alzheimer described typically began in the forties. Kraepelin concluded that it would probably turn out that we are dealing with two different conditions—one a true disease, the other a programmed disintegration related to old age.[15] Senile imbecility, in turn, had its own characteristic pathologic markers: plaques (extracellular deposits of proteinaceous material), which another scientist, Emil Redlich, had described in 1898.

Other early-twentieth-century scientists struggled with the distinction between "presenile dementia" and "senile dementia," a dichotomy that they never found entirely convincing. The American neurologist Solomon Fuller, describing a case much like Frau Auguste D. and summarizing the handful of similar cases reported in the medical literature in 1912, concluded that Alzheimer's disease was a real entity—the pathologic basis of the dementia was most likely the newly described plaques and tangles rather than atherosclerosis. But he also commented that many cases of *senile dementia* likewise demonstrated plaques without atherosclerosis. Subsequent investigators, however, typically adhered to Kraepelin's classification. They performed autopsies on elderly individuals who, they acknowledged, bore a striking resemblance in life to their younger counterparts with Alzheimer's disease.

What these scientists found on their brain examinations was exactly what they found in the presenile cases—both the plaques originally described by Redlich in old people and tangles originally described by Alzheimer in younger people. Moreover, they discovered the lesions in the same parts of the brain that were affected in Alzheimer's disease. Nonetheless, the pathologists reiterated that the two entities were different. In 1936, for example, in a paper read before the section of Nervous and Mental Diseases at the American and Canadian Medical Associations, a physician described another case like that originally presented by Alzheimer: a fifty-three-year-old with poor memory, language troubles, wandering, and difficulty dressing. At autopsy, her brain was found to be atrophic, with plaques and tangles, especially in the speech area of the brain. The author was unable to distinguish clearly between the microscopic findings in this case and in the brains of elderly individuals with dementia to which he compared them, but persisted in claiming that the plaques "somehow differ" and were perhaps more widespread with "true" Alzheimer's disease.[16]

When, in 1904, scientists isolated the spirochete, the bacterial cause of syphilis, physicians were at last able to show that some individuals with cognitive deterioration and certain psychiatric symptoms had neurosyphilis. They quickly recognized the existence of several distinct types of mental deterioration, each with a different set of symptoms and its own pathology: infection (syphilis), vascular disease (stroke), and the etiologically mysterious Alzheimer's disease. Why was it not obvious that the intellectual deterioration seen in old age was also one of these types, most commonly, Alzheimer's?[17]

Nineteenth-Century Beliefs about Old Age

It was not obvious because physicians believed that intellectual decline was part of normal aging. As one practicing physician wrote in a leading American medical journal at the turn of the century, "No sharp line can be drawn between ordinary senile dotage and senile dementia. The normal mental deterioration incident upon old age is itself early senile dementia."[18] In other words, old people lose their minds. The process is gradual, beginning with the mild symptoms characteristic of "dotage" and progressing to the more drastic symptoms of "dementia." By implication, the stages were inevitable. This perspective was common among late-nineteenth-century physicians. George Beard, for example, a distinguished American neurologist, was fascinated by aging. He had been interested in the relationship between age and creativity since his medical student days at Yale, at which time he collected data on the "greatest names in history." Beard recorded the age at which each of his idiosyncratically selected figures achieved what he deemed to be their best work, averaged the ages, and concluded that creativity peaked at forty. Using this scheme, he reasoned that 70 percent of the most original work was done by age forty-five, and 80 percent by age fifty. Putting his observations together, Beard asserted that it was "barbarian folly" to believe men could govern others when "their own brains have begun to degenerate." He spoke widely about his findings, giving lectures with such intriguing titles as "The Longevity of Brain Workers," "Legal Responsibility in Old Age," and "On the Decline of the Moral Faculties in Old Age." He went on to claim that both intellectual and moral decline were the rule in old age, leading to symptoms of querulousness, irritability, and avarice.[19]

The belief in the inevitability of age-associated cognitive decline was perfectly compatible with the view that anatomic changes accompanied mental deterioration. From the vantage point of descriptive pathology, there would of course be changes in the brain with age, and some of those—including atrophy and atherosclerosis of cerebral vessels—might be the *cause* of the expected mental deterioration. However, if dementia invariably accompanied old age, then surely the factors associated with it were different from those linked to that rare condition, "presenile dementia." This is what Ignasz Nascher, the "father of American geriatrics," argued. He wrote in his 1914 textbook: "We must look upon the degenerations, the atrophies, hypertrophies and all the changes in form and character that are due to the process of involution, as natural, normal and physiological." He explained that "senile debility is no more a pathological condition than is the weakness of the infant." He continued: "The obvious characteristics of senility are evidence in the appearance, attitude, gait, *mentality* and tout ensemble of *mental* and physical *decay.*" (Emphasis added.) He concluded: "The most profound changes occur in the function of the brain . . . the senile changes in temperament, emotion, sensations and intellect." And finally: "Of the intellectual faculties memory is usually the first to show impairment, names and numbers being quickly forgotten."[20]

The decision to maintain that Alzheimer's disease was exclusively a disease of the relatively young reflects the prejudices of turn-of-the-century society. There was nothing in the description of the symptoms or in the microscopic observations that justified a distinction between "normal" senile dementia and "abnormal" presenile dementia. The distinction was based largely on prevailing conceptions of the nature of aging.

Historians of medicine often emphasize the cultural component of science, the role of sociological and economic factors in shaping the way scientists see reality. The temptation for scientists, by contrast, is to see knowledge as monotonically increasing, moving incrementally toward the truth. Physicians are no exception: we can countenance the possibility that *what* researchers choose to study and *why* they regard certain questions as worthy of investigation are influenced by the surrounding society. But surely well-designed experiments admit of only one interpretation. And if it remains unclear what conclusions can be drawn, then the explanation is to be found in the science. Shoddy research, we tend to believe, is at the root of scientific ambiguity. But in the case of Alzheimer's disease, the problem was not poor science. Nor would the great leap in understanding depend on the discovery of a microbial cause or a definitive biochemical marker, something readily measurable through a blood test. The necessary evidence was available by 1910. Practicing physicians and clinical investigators, Americans and Europeans—none of them looked at Alzheimer's disease and senile dementia and were convinced that they were both the same disorder. They considered the possibility, but their cultural preconceptions abut aging were so powerful that ultimately they concluded that the two clinically and pathologically identical conditions were distinct.[21]

How was aging viewed one hundred years ago—what were

these strongly held beliefs about old people that implied the inevitability of intellectual deterioration with age? I had no trouble uncovering how Americans tended to see aging at the time of Alzheimer's discovery. Aging was equated with decay. Even the American geriatrician I. Nascher, revered for creating the field of geriatric medicine, had little positive to say about the elderly. His textbook, the same oeuvre that carefully distinguished between normal aging and pathologic aging, and between diseases common in old age and diseases unique to old age, had this to say about aging: "We realize that for all practical purposes the lives of the aged are useless, that they are often a burden to themselves, their family and to the community at large. Their appearance is unesthetic, their actions objectionable, their very existence often an incubus to those who in a spirit of humanity or duty take upon themselves the care of the aged." Lest there be any doubt that Nascher himself regarded his elderly patients as despicable, he went on to add: "The appearance of the senile individual is repellent both to the esthetic sense and to the sense of independence, that sense or mental attitude that the human race holds toward the self-reliant and self-dependent."[22]

Nascher's opinion was not unique. A second textbook of geriatrics, issued a few years later, echoed his sentiments. Its author, Walford Thewlis, condemned both public and medical "neglect" of the aged, and in the same breath asserted that "from the purely esthetic standpoint, the aged are disagreeable, often repulsive, repelling those whose sympathy can be aroused only by the sight of helplessness or sound of distress."[23]

Nor were negative views of aging confined to the medical profession. Even members of the pro-longevity movement (1890–1925), who sought to extend life by finding the elixir of youth, characterized aging as a disease. Precisely because old age was held to be a period of misery and misfortune, the goal of the movement was its wholesale extirpation. Only by converting old age to youth could any redeeming value be found in what was otherwise seen as a time of decline, disease, and disintegration. Indeed, the word *senile* was redefined in the nineteenth century: initially a value-neutral term meaning "old," it came to be a technical term denoting the "inevitable debilitated condition of the aged."[24]

More Positive Views of Aging and Why They Changed

Aging had not always been viewed as so unrelievedly gloomy a stage of life. In the colonial period (1620–1775), those few stalwart individuals who survived to old age were esteemed for the accomplishment. Achievement of the "senium" was taken as a mark of God's favor. The Puritans regarded all of life as a "sacred pilgrimage" culminating in death. Death, in turn, was seen as the gateway from the secular world into a holier eternal life. Not surprisingly for a society strongly influenced by biblical texts, the Puritans espoused the traditional conception of old age as a time of wisdom. Sarah, after all, gave birth to Isaac at the age of ninety. Abraham himself was said to be one hundred at the time of the birth. The claims about the ages of the patriarch and matriarch of the Jewish people strongly suggest that old age was seen as a mark of distinction.

In the late eighteenth century, old age was an intensely meaningful phase of life. It was a time to fulfill personal obligations by preparing for death. It was a time to fulfill obligations to family as well, by arranging for the division of landed property. Finally, it was a time to fulfill a responsibility to the community by serving as a source of advice and wisdom for one's neighbors. Physical decline was taken for granted in Calvinist theology, pain and chronic disease were man's punishment for the sin of Adam. The challenge of old age was to muster "the strength and courage to face one's condition openly and to fulfill final obligations."[25] Very occasionally, and for no ascertainable reason, God bestowed good health or unusual longevity on one of His creatures. Such good fortune was as unfathomable as was most misfortune: it was the positive antipode of the suffering of Job. In either case, the old person, according to the views enunciated by ministers in their sermons, was expected to make aging meaningful through piety. The model elder corresponded to the image in the New Testament: sober, pious, and patient.[26]

Over the course of the nineteenth century, this genuinely positive view of aging gradually lost its hold, in tandem with the weakening of the Calvinist worldview. The ideology of egalitarianism that emerged from the American and French Revolutions dealt the doctrine of age supremacy a heavy blow. The idea of political equality, of equality before the law, spread like wildfire throughout America, and later caught on in Europe. It radically undermined the hierarchical structure of society that accorded status to individuals based on age alone. As a result, elders were no longer given preferential seating in houses of worship, white-haired wigs were abandoned, and clothes were adopted that revealed rather than concealed. The words *gaffer* and *fogy* developed new meanings as pejorative terms for older people.[27]

Industrialization and urbanization, which followed the shift from an ideology of hierarchical communalism to one of egalitarian individualism, dealt age supremacy another blow.[28] The patriarch's power rested on his having land to bequeath, at his discretion, to his sons. When the sons lost interest in agriculture, abandoning farming for industrial jobs or to build the nation's railroads and canals, their fathers' power faded. Increasingly, society came to depend on efficiency and productivity for material progress. Not surprisingly, as capitalism replaced religion as the driving force in American society, human worth came to be defined in terms of productivity. The new ideology that developed to support the changed economic infrastructure promoted discipline and self-reliance as the primary virtues. The individual who worked hard and reined in any tendencies toward laziness or profligacy could expect to control his economic destiny. Gradually, right behavior came to be seen as the key to his spiritual and physical destiny as well.

In keeping with the cultural trend to place the responsibility—and the blame—for an individual's success in life on his own shoulders, health, disease, and ultimately aging were likewise regarded as an outgrowth of personal behavior. The health reform movement of the mid-nineteenth century was founded on precisely this concept of individual responsibility and control. Sylvester Graham (1794–1851), for instance, of graham cracker fame, emphasized the importance of diet in

maintaining health and prolonging life. Mary Gove Nichols
(1810–84) placed her faith in vegetarianism and hydropathy,
or water therapy, as the guarantors of well-being. Luther Gulick
(1865–1918), founder of the physical culture movement,
believed that regular exercise would improve both muscle
and brain power. The temperance movement focused on
alcohol as the source of ill health and abstinence as the root
of health. Other health reformers attributed illness and
physical decline to sexual excesses. In each case, the presence
of disease and dependency in old age was attributed to personal failure in the earlier years: long life and a peaceful, sudden, "natural" death were achievable through upright
living.[29]

The message that a good old age was available to all who
chose it was reinforced by nineteenth-century Protestant ministers in their sermons. Gone was the Calvinist exhortation to
transcend the miseries of old age through piety. Instead, such
preachers as Henry Ward Beecher warned that only righteous
action would lead to a good old age. The ministers of the
romantic era portrayed to their parishioners the image of the
"gentle, ripe old age of the saint" and the "nasty, disease-ridden
infirm old age of the sinner."[30]

Popular advice manuals for the elderly themselves, typically written by women, retired ministers, or sometimes physicians, reiterated the role that the individual could play in his
own health. Blaming decrepitude on past sins was probably
not well received by older people, but offering the optimistic
assurance that people could improve their lot evidently
was. Exhortations to eat well, exercise, and abstain from sex
and alcohol were consistent with the prevailing dogma of the
individual's control over his fate. The book by the physician
George Day, *A Practical Treatise on the Domestic Management and
Most Important Diseases of Advanced Life,* published in Philadelphia in 1848, devoted an entire chapter to the "hygiene of
declining life." He argued that "senile dementia is not the
universal lot of old persons, although . . . there is a general
tendency towards that state," and then claimed that mental
deterioration may be accelerated by prolonged mental exertion, too much liquor, or "venereal excesses."[31]

One difficulty with attributing healthy old age exclusively
to virtue and debilitated old age entirely to sin was that it was

clearly false. A few of the diseases of old age were unambiguously linked to the victim's earlier habits and proclivities: the dementia of syphilis could be blamed on consorting with prostitutes; the staggering gait of cerebellar ataxia could be attributed to alcohol abuse. But for many conditions afflicting the elderly, even the most fervent believers in personal responsibility were hard pressed to find a behavior to implicate. We see physicians claiming that strokes were due to excessive thinking and other physicians arguing that strokes occurred to people who failed to use their minds enough. In a ringing condemnation of the excesses he felt were at the root of apoplexy, or stroke, a physician wrote in the *Journal of the American Medical Association*: "It would be possible to pass the earthly days without apoplexy save in most rare instances, were the wisdom heeded which is gained by the knowledge that not one who has lived in violation to natural law has escaped a penalty exactly in proportion to his transgressions." He reiterated: "The number of fatalities from apoplexy would be even far greater if it were not that death claims many victims of wrong living ere the course of mistakes run by weak and deluded humanity reach the apoplectic goal." The transgressions he identified were those of the upper classes, the "thinking classes," such as coffee, alcohol, and overeating.[32] A textbook of neurology, printed at about the same time, maintained that strokes were commonly due to "intense and long-continued intellectual exertion."[33] On the other hand, the neurologist George Beard claimed that using the mind conferred longevity. While he did not specifically address the possible relationship between stroke and thinking, he insisted that the "brain-working classes," namely clergymen, lawyers, physicians, merchants, scientists, and men of letters, lived longer than the "muscle-working classes." He inveighed against those who believed that "the mind can be used only at the injurious expense of the body," a view he regarded as pernicious superstition.[34]

The late-nineteenth-century attempt to blame mental deterioration on undesirable behavior is a specific manifestation of a more general tendency to distinguish between the "worthy" and the "undeserving" elderly. Those elderly "paupers" who were presumed to have brought misery upon themselves and therefore "deserved" their status were relegated to almshouses. The gradual recognition that some poor, old people, through no fault of their own, lacked any means of support led to the development of a new institution for the care of the elderly, the old age home. Private philanthropic organizations, typically representing a specific ethnic or religious group, built facilities for the care of needy, dependent members of their community, facilities bearing less stigma than the almshouse. It is far from clear that the "unworthy poor" were any more responsible for their misfortune than their ostensibly "worthy" counterparts. Nonetheless, in the prevailing typology, individuals were held responsible for much of the adversity that befell them, whether poverty or mental deterioration.

At the same time that the model of personal culpability was breaking down, the pressures to define human worth in terms of productivity were escalating. Industrialization, which had been in its infancy in the heyday of the health reformers, was by the latter part of the nineteenth century the dominant mode of production. Progress, which had been a popular buzzword since the Enlightenment, had been refined to mean *material* progress. Post–Civil War American society was bent on making things, on extending the frontier, on finding gold in the hills. It was a society for go-getters, for entrepreneurs or, for those with less initiative or imagination, a society best suited to those willing and able to work hard in a routine job.[35] If worth was measured by output, or at least by daring, where did that leave the debilitated seventy-five-year-old with his failing eyesight, fickle joints, and fading memory?

By the end of the nineteenth century, the old person who could no longer produce was regarded as superannuated. Whether he could have prevented his decline was of little consequence and his relationship with God was a matter of indifference. The ideal man worked until the day of his death. There was simply no room in the prevailing ethos for a stage of life devoid of tangible output.

It was not very long before the bosses at the workplace recognized the need for retirement, indeed for mandatory dismissal of workers once they could no longer achieve a certain standard of production. The high probability of physical and mental decline in the elderly was a reality. Something had to be done with the old and sick: in addition to the construction of old age homes, the century witnessed the development of a professional interest in managing the needs of the elderly. But creating the field of gerontology and a cadre of specialists interested in the problems of the elderly did not ensure respect for old people. On the contrary, their dependence and lack of contribution to the gross national product guaranteed them a place of profound disrespect in the mind of the public. Charles Stephens, a popular writer at the turn of the century and an adherent of the life-extension movement, took as his starting point the belief that life was only worth prolonging if aging could be eradicated. Old age, as he saw it, was characterized by "grossness, coarseness, and ugliness." The aging body, he went on, was a "sad, strange mixture of foulness and putrefaction, in which the sweeter, purer flame of life struggles and smoulders."[36]

Popular literature had nothing good to report about old age. Henry David Thoreau (1817–62), writing in his utopian idyll, *Walden*, commented that: "I have yet to hear the first syllable of valuable or even earnest advice from my seniors. They have told me nothing and probably cannot teach me anything."[37] Walt Whitman (1819–92), in a poem written at age seventy, describes himself as "dull, parrot-like and old, with cracked voice harping, screeching."[38] Senescence was equated with decay. No longer was deterioration held to be preventable, whether by God's grace or by righteous living. The increasingly hostile attitude toward the elderly found in the writings of American literary figures, physicians, and scientists was paralleled in European society. It was not surprising that Alzheimer and his colleagues would look at dementia in a fifty-year-old and see disease, and at dementia in a seventy-year-old and see normal aging.

It is understandable why Alzheimer and Kraepelin came down in favor of distinguishing "presenile dementia" from the dementia of old age. What remains to be explained is what changed over the next fifty years that allowed old data to be interpreted in a new light. Was it a new scientific discovery or, like the views of Alzheimer and Kraepelin earlier, was the change as much a product of the prevailing attitude toward aging as it was of hard science?

The Radical Shift—the New Science

The neurologists who concluded that Alzheimer's disease was a single entity, regardless of age of onset, started with scientific facts. They looked at all the studies that had been done, which repeatedly found that the *pathology* and the *clinical course* were identical in the young and the old. Several large studies done in state mental institutions attempted to correlate clinical syndromes, observed in life, and pathologic findings, detected at death. Instead of merely reporting on one individual or summarizing the conclusions of a handful of case reports, these investigators looked at a series of consecutive patients at a single institution. They emphatically asserted that they were unable to distinguish between fifty-five-year-olds with dementia and seventy-five-year-olds with dementia either in terms of the progression of their disease or the microscopic appearance of their brains.[39]

The methods used to define "clinical syndrome" and "brain pathology" in these epidemiologic studies were crude. They allowed for the possibility that the older patients' behavior was worse, or more regressed, or their thinking more impaired than the younger patients'. They were compatible with the widespread claims that the plaques and tangles were scattered in the brain in different patterns in the two groups. To settle definitively whether Alzheimer's disease and senile dementia were really identical or whether they just appeared superficially similar, a quantitative approach was extremely helpful.

Quantitative methods in general and statistical approaches in particular had been in ascendance since World War II. They had become the dominant mode of analysis in both social science and clinical medicine by the 1960s. The limitation of the controlled scientific experiment in testing hypotheses had become painfully apparent: it simply was not possible to study people with the same degree of precision as it was to study the bacterium *Escherichia coli,* a favorite subject of experimentation. The best that could be done when investigating the effect of a new drug or other treatment in people was to randomize the patients into two groups, one that received the treatment and the other that did not. Since the subjects were arbitrarily divided into the two groups, the presumption was that any differences in outcomes could be attributed to the difference in treatment.

Quantitative methods were developed for a host of other clinical and epidemiologic problems. Hypotheses about the cause of disease, for example, could be tested by studying whether people with the disease were more likely than people without the disease to share a common exposure or a common ancestry. The link between cigarette smoking and lung cancer, for instance, was established when two British investigators used statistics rather than casual observation. They mailed questionnaires to 60,000 physicians in England, asking them about various habits and medical problems. Those who responded were followed for several years and all cases of lung cancer documented. At the end of the study period, the scientists found that the smokers' risk of developing lung cancer was *twenty-four times* that of the nonsmokers. This kind of analysis was far more persuasive than a few isolated observations suggesting that the lung from a man who died of lung cancer had characteristic changes from chronic smoking whereas the lung from a man who died at the same age of colon cancer did not.[40]

By the early 1960s, physician-scientists recognized that careful measurement allowed for far more precision than mere description. Coupled with statistics, which enabled researchers to draw conclusions about just how likely their observations were to be repeatable, and not just due to chance, the numerical approach gave investigators vast powers. This kind of quantitative thinking enabled three British investigators to shed new light on the old question of whether senile dementia and Alzheimer's disease were distinguishable. Collaborating in the town of Newcastle-on-Tyne, Martin Roth, Garry Blessed, and Bernard Tomlinson utilized three different quantitative methods. First, Blessed developed a psychological test, with questions assessing memory, language, and visuo-spatial skills. This test allowed him to measure cognitive function reproducibly, and permitted him to distinguish objectively among individuals with dementia, schizophrenia, and assorted other psychiatric disturbances. Second, Roth and Tomlinson established rigorous criteria for counting plaques and tangles in autopsy specimens. They had to specify which parts of the brain were to be examined and the dimensions of the brain slices to be looked at. Finally, they used statistical analysis to test the strength of the apparent association between the severity of the dementia and the number of plaques or tangles.[41]

The level of detail required for this kind of fastidious measurement was in turn dependent on another new technique, electron microscopy. The extraordinary magnification and resolution afforded by the electron microscope converted a mass of degenerated neurons into discrete, countable plaques. Since most elderly individuals develop plaques even if they have normal cognition, but people with Alzheimer's disease have far more plaques, it was crucial to be able to separate one plaque from the next and compute the number of plaques in a given volume of tissue (the density). This approach was unlike that used in microbiology, the study of germs, where finding just one tuberculosis bacterium in the sputum or the spinal fluid or the bone marrow clinched the diagnosis of tuberculosis. Both quantitative thinking and the reductionist view (which moved biology to ever smaller units of study—first the cell, then parts of the cell, and ultimately the molecular structure of proteins and genes) transformed American medicine in the post–World War II period.

The neuroscientists who studied Alzheimer's patients naturally looked at the problem through the spectacular lens of the electron microscope. When they sought to characterize their patients on clinical grounds, they borrowed techniques used by other scientific disciplines. Once they were ready to analyze their data, they adopted the tools their colleagues used in other pursuits. Developments in science in general clearly facilitated advances in the understanding of Alzheimer's disease. But what is not at all clear is why Blessed, Roth, Tomlinson, and a handful of others bothered to ask questions about the nature of senile dementia in the first place. Their culture and their medical training had imbued them with the conviction that cognitive decline was a normal part of growing old. Why should they have challenged this assumption?

The Radical Shift—the Role of Demography

They asked the question because something had been happening to the population that was beginning to make itself felt in physicians' offices just about the time they were conducting their research. Both Americans and Western Europeans were starting, in large numbers, to live to be very, very old.

The aging of the population had been going on for several decades. What is known as the "demographic transition" began in the United States and England in the last decade of the nineteenth century: after many years during which both fertility and mortality rates had been stable, fertility and then mortality fell dramatically. When combined with changes in migration patterns, the net result was that longevity increased *and* the fraction of the total population made up of older people increased.

The usual way of thinking about life expectancy is to measure it at birth. This approach is a misleading way of answering how old people in a society get because it is heavily influenced by the effect on longevity of infant mortality. Some demographers instead examine the average length of life achieved after reaching one's fifteenth birthday, by which time congenital abnormalities and childhood infections have done their work. Using this measure, life expectancy increased 50 percent after the demographic transition. If we look at a different statistic, the proportion of adults over sixty, a measure seeking to capture the weight of the older population, we find a 200 percent increase after the demographic transition. The rise began in the 1890s, the steepest climb occurred between 1920 and 1950, and we may, in the next century, reach a new plateau. While fluctuations in both longevity and the proportion of the population that was old occurred in previous eras, the variations tended to be small, reflecting epidemics, famines, and wars. Our ancestors never experienced aging changes on anything like the scale of the demographic transition.[42]

By the 1960s, the effects of the shift were becoming noticeable. It is not surprising that Medicare, the entitlement health insurance program for those sixty-five and over, was enacted in 1965. It is not surprising that the American Association of Retired Persons was founded in 1958 and flourished in subsequent years. The cumulative effects of the aging population hit home during the period 1940–60, when America and

Western Europe for the first time entered an era in which a large proportion of the population was composed of individuals who had retired from work or whose children had grown up and left home. Over one-fourth of all adults were over sixty and over one half of the men alive at age twenty-five were still alive at age seventy.[43]

But this change alone would not have translated into a great many more people being diagnosed with dementia, since Alzheimer's disease is relatively uncommon among sixty- to seventy-year-olds. The other startling development in the 1950s and 1960s was the rise in the number of the very old, those over eighty, or even over eighty-five. In 1900, there were 123,000 Americans eighty-five years and older, or 0.2 percent of the population. In 1940, the percentage began to rise; by 1950, there were 577,000 people eighty-five and older (0.4 percent); in 1970 the numbers jumped to 1,409,000 (0.7 percent), and in 1990, there were 3,021,000 (over 1 percent). Simply looking at how many people today are over eighty-five does not capture the magnitude of the rise. Computing the percent of the total population who are eighty-five and over likewise does not highlight the change, because the percentages are still small. If we create a new measure, the fraction of the elderly population (all those sixty-five and over) who are at least eighty-five, what we find is that this number began a sharp ascent in 1950 and has been soaring ever since. With a little dip when the baby boomers reach sixty-five (the percent of the elderly population who are over eighty-five will fall as the total elderly population balloons) and then a big jump when the baby boomers reach eighty-five, the percentage rises from a constant 4 percent until 1950 to a staggering 24 percent projected by 2050.

For researchers in the 1950s and 1960s, the new demographic reality must have had a palpable effect: suddenly they were seeing a great many octogenarians in their offices and in the hospital. Between one quarter and one half of these very old people were demented. Far from being a rare condition, or one that afflicted the handful of people who survived to very old age, dementia was popping up everywhere.

For some of the neuroscientists who chose to concentrate their professional energies on Alzheimer's disease, it had invaded their personal lives as well. Robert Katzman was a young neurologist who, in the late 1950s, worked in a laboratory at the Albert Einstein College of Medicine in New York. He was on his way to becoming a successful scientist—which meant publishing papers, obtaining grants, and eventually establishing his own laboratory. The usual pathway for an ambitious young researcher is to apprentice himself to a senior scientist in order to learn the techniques needed for experimentation, to carve out his own niche within or related to his mentor's area of interest. Katzman did exactly that, working under the direction of Saul Korey, a neurologist and neurochemist who was interested in a number of degenerative brain diseases, including Alzheimer's.

To his surprise, Dr. Katzman found that many of the brain biopsies he performed on patients suspected of having a variety of fairly rare forms of dementia proved that the patients in fact had something else—they had the characteristic plaques and tangles of Alzheimer's disease. At the same time, his mother-in-law was diagnosed with Alzheimer's disease. As Katzman looked at the deterioration of his wife's previously vibrant mother, he could not believe that what she had was simply normal aging. But if her cognitive decline was not normal, then neither was the dementia that he was seeing all around him in his professional life, 50 to 60 percent of which he estimated to be of the Alzheimer's type. A terrible disease was making its way through the elderly population— in epidemic proportions.

Driven by both domestic and demographic realities, Katzman came to the conclusion that the phrase *senile dementia* should be replaced by more precise terms—*Alzheimer's disease* or *multi-infarct dementia* or *normal pressure hydrocephalus*—all various forms of the disorder dementia. He also concluded that what came to be known as "senile dementia of the Alzheimer's type" and eventually simply as Alzheimer's disease indirectly caused a large fraction of deaths in the elderly. Dementia can be said to be the cause of death because it predisposes its victims to pneumonia and blood clots to the lungs, and perhaps to strokes and heart attacks. He estimated that even though Alzheimer's disease scarcely ever appeared on death certificates as the cause of death, it was in fact the fourth leading cause among the elderly.

The inference that Alzheimer's disease in younger people

and in older people was indistinguishable was based on scientific observation; the proclamation that Alzheimer's was a disease, regardless of age of onset, was a matter of interpretation. Katzman could equally well have concluded that dementia, with plaques and tangles in the brain, was the *usual* concomitant of aging. He might have reasoned that a few unfortunate individuals developed the syndrome early and a fair number survived into their eighties and nineties without cognitive deterioration, but that dementia, like gray hair or farsightedness, was a characteristic feature of aging.

There is ample precedent for identifying phenomena that steadily rise in frequency with aging as *diseases*. High blood pressure also increases dramatically with age. Two-thirds of individuals over the age of sixty-five have some form of high blood pressure.[44] Simply redefining what was normal blood pressure in older people proved to be problematic as evidence accumulated that the high blood pressure of old people predisposed them to strokes and heart attacks. Statistically speaking, the blood pressure changes were normal, but from a clinical perspective they were devastating. For years, physicians clung to the belief that only diastolic hypertension—the elevation of the second number in the blood pressure measurement, the pressure generated in the blood vessels between cardiac contractions, when the heart muscle was at rest—was related to the development of strokes and heart attacks. Diastolic hypertension, as well as combined systolic and diastolic hypertension, were the forms of blood pressure abnormality commonly seen in middle-aged people. Isolated systolic hypertension—the exclusive elevation of the first number in the blood pressure measurement, the maximum pressure produced during cardiac contraction—was the kind of blood pressure change found commonly and almost exclusively in older people. Surely this kind of blood pressure alteration was just a normal part of aging, attributable to hardening of the arteries. But large studies in many Western nations confirmed that isolated systolic hypertension, too, is associated with strokes and heart attacks—in fact to an even greater degree than diastolic hypertension. Moreover, the evidence mounted from intervention trials that treatment of systolic hypertension with medication substantially reduces the rate of both heart attacks and strokes.

From a strictly medical point of view—as opposed to a social or political or philosophical point of view—whether Alzheimer's disease is viewed as more like pneumonia, hypertension, or farsightedness is of little import. It does not matter whether it is unambiguously a disease (like pneumonia), which strikes a limited number of people and is due to an infectious agent; or whether it is a characteristic that rises in prevalence with age (like hypertension), that in turn causes other diseases, and which is amenable to treatment or prevention; or whether it is an invariable concomitant of aging (like farsightedness) that can nonetheless be compensated for. All three types of conditions can be described and analyzed, diagnosed and treated, and sometimes obliterated.

The psychological reality confronting neuroscientists such as Katzman, however, was that old people with dementia appeared to be transformed. Eighty-year-olds without dementia, by contrast, clearly had the same personality, the same likes and dislikes, as their younger selves.[45] To regard dementia as a normal part of aging when it apparently undermined continuity with the earlier self was difficult to accept. From this perspective—and not merely because of the lessons of hard science—it made sense to consider "senile dementia" and "presenile dementia" as identical. The most common form of dementia was Alzheimer's disease, which was presumed to have a cause and a cure—if only we can find them.

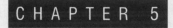

CHAPTER 5

Evening Star

Perhaps if Sylvia Truman had grown up in an era when day care for children was commonplace, she would have been more favorably disposed toward the adult day program she attended. Alternatively, she might have been even more hostile, asserting peremptorily that day care was for toddlers, not doddering old women. As it was, she had no preconceived notions about day care, either the pediatric or the geriatric variety. She had not liked the concept of a structured activities center, preferring to be left to her own devices, and the reality proved even less appealing.

The program Sylvia went to was a superb representative of the genre. I routinely took medical students to visit during their few weeks studying geriatrics. Sometimes I checked on patients while they were in day care instead of trying to orchestrate an office visit—to come to the office would disrupt their entire day. They would probably miss day care entirely, since they typically relied on a van to transport them to and from home. Someone would need to bring them to see me, most likely a family member who would have to take off a day of work to accompany them and then stay with them afterwards. For me to go to the day care center was comparatively easy: Park Valley Day Center was only a few minutes' drive from the hospital where I worked and, with luck, I might have several patients there simultaneously. Since the visits with medical students had been a success, and since I had to pay a call on Louise Callahan, recently discharged after a mild heart attack, I decided to drop in together with one of the hospital interns.

The center was in a large, airy room on the ground level of a church. All the action took place in the main room, though there was a kitchen off to one side where the director refrigerated the participants' medications and prepared their lunches and snacks. Another small room served as the nurse's office, equipped with basic supplies such as a blood pressure cuff, a scale, and first aid materials. Anne McPherson, nurse, director, social worker, and recreation therapist rolled into one, greeted us when we arrived. She saw the skeptical expression on my younger colleague's face and immediately seized the opportunity to proselytize.

Anne McPherson was a woman with a mission. She believed that adult day care, when done right, could do far more than just keep frail old people out of nursing homes—though that in itself was a laudable goal. She felt that day care could rescue people who were lonely and bored by offering them companionship and meaningful activities. She aspired to create a therapeutic milieu at her center, stamping out the sense of despair and worthlessness that sent so many older people sliding into a state of depression. Anne McPherson was ambitious for herself and for the center. She also loved her work and the twenty-five elderly people who came to the center. She knew them all—their likes and dislikes, their quirks and their talents, their medical problems and their families. She showed us how she had taken the one large room and divided it into four cozier activity areas, some with tables and chairs, another with lounge chairs and a sofa. Instead of decorating the walls with the current artwork of her charges, which would regrettably have given the place the appearance of a nursery school, she had asked everyone to bring in a framed photograph. A few of the women still did needlepoint, and their handiwork was prominently displayed as well.

"Come look around," the director commanded. "You're here to see Louise? She's busy right now, playing poker. You can't possibly interrupt her." I thought of the nursing homes I visited, where my patients were routinely taken away from whatever they were doing for my convenience. Here, the priorities were clear-cut: a physician visit was not the most important or exciting part of the day. "You can't imagine what I had to go through to get permission from the church to hold a poker game here. They've otherwise been very accommodating, but they were firm on this one. Poker is gambling and gambling is not allowed. But I argued that the church has a bingo game on the premises every month, and they play for *money*. My people don't play for money. And they're not playing strip poker!" Then she added softly, "Though we have had a few romances here." She gestured to the sofa where a handsome silver-haired man was holding hands with a diminutive older woman, her back bent from osteoporosis, hearing aids in both ears, wearing thick cataract glasses. "Dora's doctor advised her to have a lens implant— she had her cataracts removed ages ago, before they did lens implants, so she has those old-fashioned glasses. The arthritis in her hands is so bad that she can't possibly deal with contact lenses that you put in and take out. But Dora just looked at the doctor and told him her boyfriend didn't mind her glasses, and the doctor was so surprised he didn't know what to say. They met here, Dora and Frank. Both live alone in different apartment buildings for the elderly. They like to sit together and listen to popular music from the thirties." She pointed to the tape player on the coffee table in front of them. "If you have any old records, give them to me and I'll tape them for our collection."

The young doctor who was with me had not wanted to visit an adult day care center. He was much more comfortable on his own turf, in the hospital, preferably in the intensive care unit, with lab test results to ponder and procedures to do. But he was taken with Frank and Dora in spite of himself. "I hope when I'm old I have a girlfriend who looks at me that way," he commented. I wondered how many people his age had partners who were as mutually accepting and devoted as Frank and Dora, let alone how many octogenarians.

"We do have some arts and crafts," Miss McPherson continued, propelling us toward a table where a half dozen old women were making artificial flowers to plant in genuine flower pots. "Lots of senior centers give their old people watercolors or crayons and treat them as though they were three years old. My philosophy is that art projects are fine if they are meaningful to the person doing them. Those flowers that Lucinda is making"—she pointed to a sprig of very realistic-appearing daisies—"will brighten up her bedroom. They won't shrivel up and die, and she won't have to water them, either. And the knitting that some of my ladies do!" She marched over to a woman with a parkinsonian tremor who was struggling to knit. "This is Georgia Canaby. She's *amazing!*" Mrs. Canaby blushed. "She's making a sweater for her great-grandson. Now that's something his parents will really appreciate, and it's much better quality than those synthetic things in the stores." We followed Miss McPherson to the nurse's office, passing the last cluster of people, who were seated in a semicircle, listening with varying degrees of attention as a staff member read aloud from the newspaper. "Some of my ladies don't have the cognitive capacity to make anything useful or pretty, at least not on their own. Everyone likes to eat, though, and most of them used to do all the cooking. So with a lot of supervision, they can participate in a cooking project. I always try to get a group together to make one of the lunch dishes." I noticed Sylvia Truman among the women in the news group. She was fidgeting with her dress. "That's one of my newest," Miss McPherson commented, following my gaze. "She doesn't want to be here. She wants to believe she doesn't belong because she's in better shape than the others. Even after she fell and broke her hip she believed she was perfectly healthy. Actually, she is in reasonably good physical condition, but cognitively she's among the less intact. Not as bad as Mary over there." She nodded in the direction of one woman who was pacing back and forth. "*She's* a real problem. I've tried everything to soothe her, to make her less anxious—different kinds of music, games, movies. Nothing works. I'm going to have to ask that her doctor order some medication or she won't be able to come here anymore." From her tone of voice, this was clearly a mark of failure. "Louise is finished with her game. You can bring her to the office and check her now."

I introduced the intern I was with to Louise Callahan. We did our doctorly work in the back room—Louise was in remarkably good shape—and said our good-byes to Anne McPherson. "You should really stay for my reminiscence group. It's the best part of the day. Even those who are losing touch with the present usually remember phenomenal things about the past. I've learned about New York in the nineteen twenties and what the Depression was like—you'd be astonished how many people say they remember just what they were doing when they heard the stock market crashed. I'm recording our sessions and hope to interest a graduate student in an oral history project. We're making books to pass on to the grandchildren. And talking about the past helps the group remember who they are and to feel positive about themselves even in the face of decline and disability. I wish Sylvia Truman would open up and participate."[1] I wished she would, too. Anne McPherson was an extraordinary woman—energetic, creative, knowledgeable, and tremendously caring. If she could not reach Sylvia, I doubted anyone could.

Sylvia was not thriving in day care and she was not thriving at home. Moreover, although she did not recall the night spent on the bathroom floor, her son and daughter-in-law did. They jumped whenever the telephone rang, half expecting news of another disaster. They still felt guilty, as though lack of vigilance on their part had led to Sylvia's fracture. They regretted their missed vacation, and felt they could never go away unless Sylvia lived somewhere with on-site supervision.

The Truman family met with Nancy Kingsley, my social work colleague, to discuss alternative living situations. They knew Sylvia would not be pleased, but they were unanimous that the time had come for her to move. One possibility was a rest home, or board and care facility. These are not technically nursing homes, as they do not fall under the same bureaucratic jurisdiction as conventional nursing homes, nor is the tab at such facilities paid by Medicaid, as it is in full-fledged nursing homes, where those who are impoverished are eligible for Medicaid. A typical rest home is a converted old mansion with a communal dining room, a large living room, and small private rooms to accommodate a total of fifteen to fifty individuals. One nurse—usually a licensed practical nurse rather than the more highly trained registered nurse—is on duty at least eight hours a day, and in some facilities around the clock. She is available to check blood pressures, dispense medications to those few residents unable to remember their pill-taking regimens, and to make a preliminary assessment if a resident becomes acutely ill. Meals are provided, as is once-a-week housekeeping. There are few regularly scheduled activities, as most of the tenants are sufficiently vigorous to go out on their own: they simply want the company afforded by a residential community and wish to avoid the burdens of housekeeping.[2]

The newest option is assisted living, a modified version of the board and care home that has existed since the nineteenth century. The developers of assisted living saw a market niche in an as yet scarcely regulated form of care for the elderly—an institution for people who need only a minimum of help with their activities of daily living. The typical assisted living facility is made up of one-bedroom apartments, with a few studios and an occasional two-bedroom for a couple or for siblings; each apartment has its own limited kitchen facilities, a bathroom, and a small living room. The building encourages socialization through a communal dining room—required for at least one meal, available for all three, and mandatory for all three at some sites. There are also activity rooms and spacious living rooms to facilitate interaction among the residents. Associated with the assisted living complex are typically an activities director, who organizes concerts, movies, lectures, and other special programs, and a van to take the residents shopping or to medical appointments. Aides are available to provide personal care to each resident several hours a week—enough time to assist regularly with showering and dressing.

The major drawback to assisted living is that it uproots the individual from his home, transplanting him to a foreign environment, often in a different neighborhood—in some instances to a new state, so as to be closer to his children—typically among strangers. A second potential problem is that the quality of the services provided, the food, the activities, the personal assistance, are dependent on the management and are highly variable. Finally, assisted living is expensive. It is not covered by Medicaid, which pays for nursing homes for those with low incomes and few assets. It is not covered by Medicare, which pays only for short-term nursing home stays if skilled nursing is required on a daily basis. Prices vary

tremendously—by geographic area, by services provided—
but in the Boston area, where Sylvia Truman lived, the minimum was $2,500 a month.

"Which isn't bad," John Truman observed, calculating
rapidly. "That includes heat and electricity, local telephone
calls, once-a-week housekeeping, and three full meals a day—
served by waitresses. Plus the personal care and the activities.
We've already gotten rid of the car, but for many people,
moving into a place like this means they can sell their car."

"I think we ought to move her now, while she can still
enjoy some degree of independence," Marcia agreed at their
meeting with the social worker. It was settled quickly. Sylvia
visited two buildings in her area and agreed on the one that
was closer to John and Cynthia. She was less than enthusiastic
but nonetheless accepting. Perhaps she was resigned to the
need for a change and regarded this alternative as less odious
than what she had feared. On some level she knew that the
current system was marginal—she did not like the day care
program, she didn't like her housekeeper's cooking, and
despite her protestations to the contrary, she was lonely.

The first month in her new home was rough, John reported in a chance encounter as he waited for the elevator in
my office building, on the way to see his own physician. One
of the children called every morning at seven to make sure
Sylvia was awake and getting ready for breakfast. When they
called, she had sometimes been up for hours, uncertain as to
where she was or what she was expected to do. On other occasions, she thought it was seven in the evening and that she
ought to be preparing for bed. But on most days she was up,
had taken a shower on her own, and was waiting first for their
call, then for the clock to say 7:30, which meant the dining
room would be open for breakfast. Sylvia's apartment was on
the fourth floor, adjacent to the elevator so she could find it
easily. When she reached the ground floor, she often had difficulty locating the dining room. On one family visit, when
she had proudly marched her entire clan down the hall in the
wrong direction, she announced firmly that "the management moved the dining room again." But many of the other
tenants were as easily disoriented. The real question was how

long the quasi-institutional setting would provide sufficient supervision for Sylvia Truman.

That was the question John and Cynthia wanted answered when they brought Sylvia to see me three months after she had moved into her new surroundings. More precisely, they were eager to have her take an experimental drug that offered some chance of slowing the progression of Alzheimer's disease. They wanted to maintain her quality of life—which currently was borderline tolerable but was destined to become unacceptably low if she experienced further deterioration. A major determinant of quality was where she lived. A move to a nursing home, which was where she was headed next, would, they felt, dramatically change Sylvia's life for the worse. Institutionalization would reduce her privacy and further shrink her already reduced sense of independence. If medication held out the possibility of preserving the status quo, even for six months, they were interested in trying it.

I asked Sylvia how she was feeling. "Fine," she answered with a blandness that suggested otherwise.

"How's living in your new apartment?" I tried.

This elicited a more venomous response. "It's no good. It's not my home. I feel like I'm in a foreign country."

Her answer pained her daughter-in-law. "But Mom, you have your own furniture—all the things you used in the old house. And we fixed it up with your favorite prints and photographs. It's a lot cheerier than your house was: there's so much sun and the wallpaper isn't that horrid flowery stuff—"

"I liked my wallpaper," Sylvia interrupted. "And it doesn't do any good that I have my own furniture. Everything's in the wrong place so I can't find anything."

"It takes a while to adjust to such a major change," I sympathized. "Lots of new faces, too. Have you made any new friends?"

"The people there aren't like me. They're all so *old*. Lots of them use those, those things they lean on."

"You mean canes?"

"Yes, canes. They use canes and some of them have chairs, those special chairs. . . ." Her voice faded away as she struggled to find the word.

"Wheelchairs?"

"That's right. Everyone is at least eighty."

"And how old are you, Mom?" John broke in.

"Me? I'm about seventy-nine."

"Actually you just had a birthday. Remember we all went out to dinner together? To that new Italian place that just opened? You turned eighty-four."

"Did I?" Sylvia was surprised. "Well, I'm in much better shape than most of the people at that place you found for me. And their memories! They tell the same stories over and over, and all they care about is the food." Cynthia repressed a laugh.

"How is the food?"

"No good. That is, it's not, it's not what I . . ." Again she searched the unyielding recesses of her memory.

"It's not the kind of food you're used to," John supplied. He looked pained, both at her manifest dissatisfaction with the new home he had worked assiduously to choose for her, and with her increasing difficulty in word finding. "Mom's background is Italian, and she used to make extraordinary pasta. We grew up on manicotti and ravioli and lasagna—all homemade. I guess it shows." He smiled and patted his generous midriff.

"They have 'Italian night' once a week." Sylvia radiated disdain. "And they don't have any choice. It's not a restaurant," she protested.

"They do have choice," Cynthia interjected defensively. She also was having a hard time letting Sylvia attack the facility. "But they have only two choices for each meal. Usually you like one of the selections, don't you, Mom?" she wheedled.

"Usually. This morning, though, you should have seen what they did at breakfast. They ran out of orange juice! Imagine that! I had to have . . ." She paused as she stumbled over the word and then, when she could not find what she was looking for, finished meekly: "I had to have something else."

John and I smiled at Sylvia's preserved sense of outrage. I think he was pleased that the gravest sin to date appeared to be running out of orange juice, which he clearly regarded as forgivable. For Cynthia, her mother-in-law's virulence was too much to bear. "Had they ever run out of orange juice before, Mom?"

"No, not that I can recall. They might have."

"And how long have you lived in the new building?" Cynthia persisted.

"Oh, about a month."

"No," Cynthia continued triumphantly. "It's been three months. Three months and one week. I think running out of orange juice once in three months isn't so bad. I run out of orange juice at home every so often."

Sylvia bent her head slightly and averted Cynthia's gaze. She was hurt, embarrassed by the public disclosure of her forgetfulness. "Well, I never ran out of orange juice when I was bringing up my family," she managed to fire back.

I decided we had heard enough about the assisted living facility; it was time to move on to the question of medication. There had been a connection—I hadn't merely been making polite conversation. I had wanted to determine whether Sylvia Truman showed signs of depression in addition to her dementia. When I had first met her, the psychiatrist had felt strongly that her forgetfulness, her poor judgment, her difficulty finding her way were all pure manifestations of dementia. There had been nothing to point to depression: no trouble sleeping, no diminished appetite, no feelings of guilt or hopelessness. With the progression of her disease, however, Sylvia had come to sense her limitations. She denied that she had anything more than a mild memory problem, acceptable for someone her age; she insisted she was far better off than the other tenants of the assisted living complex—but at the same time she implicitly recognized that she had to be in a protected environment. She disparaged the food but acknowledged that it was awfully nice not to have to shop and cook for herself, or to rely on a housekeeper whose culinary skills were even more deplorable than those of her new community's chef. She complained about the limited range of shopping opportunities offered by the building's van service but no longer mentioned driving herself.

The awareness of dependency often brings depression in its wake. Depression can easily be mistaken for an exacerbation of the underlying dementia, which can also produce apathy and disinterest. Often I prescribe antidepressant medication to determine if a component of the listlessness is indeed depression by seeing whether it responds to treatment. I would have liked to have had a straightforward test for depression, but no blood test or X ray could reveal the patient's emotional state.

The Sylvia Truman who sat in my office to discuss experimental treatment for Alzheimer's disease was negative about her new surroundings and was saddened by her recent losses—of her home, her independence. But her sadness struck me as appropriate: she did not spend her days crying or otherwise mourning the person she had once been. When she awoke at five in the morning, hers was not the sleeplessness of the morbidly miserable but rather the result of going to bed too early compounded by an afternoon nap. The treatment for her mild but pervasive dissatisfaction with her life was engagement in more activities, not an antidepressant medication like Prozac or its cousins Zoloft and Paxil. This is not to downplay the boon sometimes provided by these drugs. In the right patient, under the right circumstances, they could vastly improve quality of life. Their predecessors in the pharmacological realm, the tricyclic antidepressants (drugs such as amitriptyline, nortriptyline, and desipramine, better known by their brand names Elavil, Pamelor, and Norpramin) were likewise remarkable chemicals, but were apt to cause confusion, sedation, or dizziness in older individuals— particularly Elavil. Sylvia, my notes reminded me, had been on an antidepressant prior to her initial geriatric consultation. At the time, its only effects had been a dry mouth and possibly a worsening of Sylvia's confusion. I thought that antidepressant medication was equally unlikely to be helpful to Sylvia now.

That was unfortunate, as the only other medications approved by the Food and Drug Administration specifically for use in Alzheimer's disease were two controversial drugs, tacrine and its cousin donepezil. "Before thinking about experimental drugs," I suggested, "let's talk about other agents approved for use in dementia." Sylvia stared at me blankly, evidently not making the connection between dementia and herself.

Cynthia went on the attack. "You didn't suggest any medication when we first brought Mom to you."

"Most of the neurologists and other geriatricians I know

and work with feel these are poor drugs that don't work very well and are expensive; tacrine at least has significant side effects. Donepezil seems to have fewer side effects, but it was approved by the FDA based on very limited studies."

"It sounds as though you didn't recommend them because you don't have stock in the companies that make them," John joked, coming to my rescue. "But maybe you should tell us a little more about these drugs."

"The idea behind both tacrine and donepezil is that people with Alzheimer's disease don't have enough of the neurotransmitter acetylcholine in their brains. And we can't simply give people acetylcholine in pill form because the chemical would be broken down in the bloodstream long before it reached the brain. What tacrine does, by contrast, is to prevent the destruction of acetylcholine—basically it allows the neurotransmitter that is present in the brain, and there is some, to last longer. Donepezil works the same way. So far there have been several controlled studies of tacrine, studies in which some patients took the drug and other comparable patients took a placebo without the doctor or the patient knowing whether he was getting tacrine or not. The studies show that tacrine produces a measurable effect—there is a slight but statistically significant increase in the scores on several neuropsychological tests in people taking tacrine, at least if they take a sufficiently high dose. But it's less clear that the improvement in test scores translates into any meaningful improvement in daily functioning. And it's very clear that about a third of patients who take high doses of tacrine, the amount needed for it to work, develop liver toxicity." Cynthia looked appalled. I hastened to assure her: "The liver changes are entirely reversible: it's just a matter of monitoring the liver with frequent blood tests, and if the enzymes normally made by the liver rise dramatically, indicating liver inflammation, then the tacrine has to be stopped and the liver tests revert to normal." I waited for all that to sink in.[3]

"And that other drug, donepezil?"

"Same story, but it does not seem to have the same problem of liver toxicity. It also can be taken just once a day instead of four times a day."

"Well, Ma, what do you say? Do you want to try some?" John asked. Cynthia was startled. She obviously had concluded that she and John were now the decision makers for Sylvia. Sylvia tacitly agreed. She shrugged. "Whatever you think."

"Gee, Ma, I thought you might help me out on this one." Sylvia looked befuddled. John chuckled. I saw he was struggling with what to decide. He turned to me. "So what do you recommend? What would you do if it were your mother?"

I was often asked that question. It was a tricky one, because my willingness to take risks, or my mother's willingness to take risks, might be quite different from my patient's. I might personally find Alzheimer's disease so awful, its slow destruction of mind and personality so devastating, that I would take any medication, however toxic, if it held some promise for improvement, however small. I had patients for whom Alzheimer's disease, while hardly a blessing, was accepted along with their high blood pressure and arthritis and glaucoma. It was "old-timer's disease," one of the perils of growing old. For other patients, the personality changes exerted a calming effect: they seemed to mellow rather than becoming anxious or depressed as they lost their bearings in the world. To ask what I would recommend for someone close to me was a little unfair. I decided that what John really wanted to know was what I recommended for Sylvia, given what I knew about her.

"I think these drugs do little if anything. They're expensive—a month of donepezil costs about $137—and potentially harmful. I don't usually recommend them to my patients, but if someone wants to try, I don't have a problem with that. And you should know that there is one article that claims that people who take fairly high doses of tacrine stay out of nursing homes longer than people who take lower doses or no medication.[4]

"There's another possibility, something that isn't exactly experimental but that hasn't been approved for use in Alzheimer's disease yet: vitamin E. A major multicenter study suggested that people taking vitamin E or another related drug, selegeline, stayed out of nursing homes longer. Vitamin E is an anti-oxidant, and some scientists think it might help prevent damage to neurons from whatever causes the injury to neurons in Alzheimer's disease."[5]

"So what horrible things does vitamin E do?" John asked, having learned to be suspicious of most medication.

"In low doses, probably nothing. In high doses, such as the dose used in the study, it can cause bleeding problems."

"Why don't we give Mom a little bit of vitamin E?"

I agreed that his suggestion would be reasonable, but I pointed out that it was far from clear that vitamin E in high doses was truly effective, and there was even less reason to believe it worked in lower doses.

"If Mom tries it and it doesn't help, are there any research drugs out there?"

I told the Trumans about one promising-sounding protocol: a study was under way at a major nearby hospital to test the efficacy of another drug in slowing the progression of mild to moderate Alzheimer's disease. I rummaged through my filing cabinet and found a letter soliciting referrals from primary care physicians, geriatricians, and neurologists. The investigators sought individuals who were otherwise in good health and who had never taken other medications purporting to ameliorate the symptoms of dementia. In fact, it looked from the description as though patients could not be taking antipsychotic medication, such as the Haldol Sylvia still took once a day, while enrolled in the study. The neurologists doing the research would administer an extensive battery of tests—including a head CAT scan and detailed neuropsychological tests. They would repeat the neuropsychological tests (which took about three hours) at six-week intervals. During the interim, they would monitor drug levels with periodic blood tests. Enrollment would mean a trip to the hospital every three weeks, with alternate short visits (for blood tests and a caregiver questionnaire) and longer visits (for the formal testing). The experimental drug was free. Because the subjects were randomized to a test group and a control group, there was a 50 percent chance that Sylvia would receive the active medication and an equal chance that her free drug would be a placebo.

"I don't want to go back and forth to any hospital for more tests," Sylvia declared. "I've already had plenty of tests, and they've come out fine."

Cynthia's lips straightened resolutely. "Perhaps we'd better think about this at home."

"I don't need to think anymore. I don't want any pills. I don't need them. And I especially don't want any tests." The old Sylvia glimmered briefly: the strong-willed, opinionated, confident Sylvia. As her memory failed, her reasoning declined, and her judgment wavered, she had become far more uncertain, more tentative in her views, if she had any at all. But she felt strongly about the issue of experimental medication, and she managed to find the words to express her feelings.

The trouble was that Sylvia no longer possessed the capacity to think about the consequences of her actions. She was worried about the here and now—taking the pills, going into the hospital to be prodded, measured, queried; her family was worried about what would happen to her in six months or a year. If she did not try a new medication, if she did not put up with the indignities and inconvenience of participation in a study protocol, was she not guaranteed to need a nursing home in the near future? Was a drug against dementia not her only hope for postponing what was otherwise inevitable?

Research in demented subjects is a perilous but essential undertaking. Testing medication is problematic because the subject typically cannot grasp all the implications of enrollment in a study—the benefits as well as the risks. Medications that offer the possibility of alleviating the suffering of the person who takes it are often worth the potential side effects if the disease is dreadful and if there is no established treatment. But what about new, ostensibly improved sleeping pills and antidepressants and antiulcer medications? Their efficacy and safety warrant testing, and just because they are well tolerated in otherwise healthy young people or in vigorous older individuals does not ensure that they will not produce increased confusion or lethargy in elderly persons with Alzheimer's disease. And there are already sleeping pills, antidepressants, and medications against ulcers with known success rates and known side effects. Is it reasonable for a demented patient with insomnia or depression or peptic ulcer disease to be enrolled in a study testing a new medication instead of simply taking an existing preparation?

Most family members of Alzheimer's disease patients are quite risk averse when it comes to authorizing experimental therapy for their charges. Unless the prevailing treatment is extremely noxious and the study drug purportedly free of side effects, family members are usually hesitant to give permission to try the new therapy. Alternatively, if the standard approach is only minimally effective and the improved version claims a far higher cure rate, the patient's surrogate decision maker might be willing to approve a trial of the new treatment.

When cognitively intact older individuals are asked whether, if they become demented, they would be willing to be the subjects of medical research, a large percentage assent. They hope to better their own condition and to be of service to others by their participation. But these same people seldom advise their spouses or adult children of their views, so the conservative strategy of the family prevails. As a result, few demented elderly enter research protocols. Data about the risks and benefits of new therapies must be extrapolated from younger, healthier patients, with the result that any side effects of such drugs that are found exclusively in those with cognitive impairment are often unappreciated until long after the medication has been on the market.

To afford more individuals with Alzheimer's disease the opportunity to be part of a clinical investigation, the elderly should be encouraged to complete advance directives authorizing their health care proxies to enroll them in studies if they lose the capacity to sign themselves up. Ideally, families should be educated about the importance of randomized trials to guide future therapy, and made aware of the extent to which many people are eager for the chance to be of help to others.[6]

I got a call from John Truman that his mother remained adamant that she wanted no more testing and did not feel she needed any medication. "Does she remember the conversation we had?" I asked, somewhat doubtful.

"No. Each time I bring it up, we have to start from the beginning again. But she's very consistent. Whenever I tell her why she should try the new medication she says no. And when I tell her why it's worth putting up with a few tests, she says no. Her reaction is always the same: she feels fine and doesn't want pills. In fact, she stopped taking her Haldol. Then she says she's had plenty of tests—and none of them have done her any good. I can't see trying to make her go along with something she opposes, although it is frustrating because she doesn't understand what's in store for her and how medicine might help stave off that future. As it is, it will be a battle to get her to take her blood pressure medicine."

I had to agree. If the pills in question offered the possibility of curing Alzheimer's disease (if the potential benefit were great), and if the only drawback were the inconvenience of traveling to the hospital for tests (if the burden were small), then it would make sense to cajole, coax, and perhaps even coerce Sylvia into trying the proposed pills. For now, I had to admit that while Sylvia's capacity to make decisions was limited, she retained the ability to understand the issue at hand and her choice was clear: she would remain in the assisted living complex as long as her function permitted, taking only her blood pressure medication. The Truman family would have to be content with the status quo and await a new crisis in Sylvia's life.

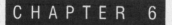

CHAPTER 6

Alzheimer's Disease— the Politics

Already when she first came to see me, Sylvia Truman's world had shrunk to her immediate neighborhood. She could no longer process global politics: she could not imagine other peoples in distant lands and, as her dementia progressed, her sense of time and place became increasingly distorted. Sylvia could grasp that I believed there was something wrong with her memory—though she thought I was wrong. But the politics of Alzheimer's were completely beyond her. Nonetheless, politics is the engine behind the mammoth research effort that has made considerable progress in understanding Alzheimer's and promises much more in the future; politics is the basis of the strong lobbying group dedicated to promoting the very interests that Sylvia does not know she has.

The Politicization of Alzheimer's Disease

By the 1970s, those few medical scientists who thought about dementia were increasingly convinced that the distinction between "presenile" and "senile" forms was artificial. Dementia was dementia, regardless of the age of onset. It was a syndrome, a collection of symptoms with a variety of possible causes. The principle cause—whether in people in their fifties and sixties, or in their seventies and eighties—was Alzheimer's disease. Recognizing that Alzheimer's was something other than an obscure neurologic disorder was the first step in achieving status in the medical arena. But for Alzheimer's to become a household word, and for it to attract millions of dollars in research grants, more was needed. Alzheimer's was catapulted into prominence because of a conscious *political* decision. The politicization of Alzheimer's disease was a multifaceted process that started with the public portrayal of the disease as a public health disaster.

At a conference of neurologists meeting in Houston in 1979, and then in an editorial published in the *Archives of Neurology* two years later, the distinguished neuroscientist Robert Katzman asserted that Alzheimer's disease was far more common than was widely believed. It afflicted approximately 1 million Americans and moreover, it was "malignant," killing between sixty thousand and ninety thousand people each year. He concluded that "in focusing attention on the mortality associated with Alzheimer disease, our goal is not to find a way to prolong the life of severely demented persons, but rather to call attention to our belief that senile as well as presenile forms of Alzheimer are a single disease, a disease whose etiology must be determined, whose course must be aborted, and ultimately a disease to be prevented."[1]

Simply bringing a problem to the attention of his professional colleagues did not, of course, ensure either that the matter would be taken seriously or that his concern would be acted upon. Moreover, Katzman's call to action took the form of an editorial rather than a sober, scientific paper reporting a breakthrough. The significance of Katzman's warning was amplified because, at the very same time, another movement was afoot. This movement, which would have dramatic consequences for the future of research on Alzheimer's disease, consisted of a push to form a separate institute on aging within the National Institutes of Health.

The National Institutes of Health (NIH) had, since World War II, been the major source of funding for biomedical research in the United States. First established as the National Institute (singular) of Health in 1930, it was a small operation until it moved to a large, privately donated estate in Bethesda in 1938. At just about that time, Congress passed legislation establishing a separate unit, the National Cancer Institute, under the aegis of the NIH. Congress also empowered the

Public Health Service to award grants to researchers working in laboratories off the NIH campus and to fund training fellowships in medical research. The NIH at the end of World War II was itself a small organization with a research budget of $180,000. But the successes of targeted medical research during the war, exemplified by the development and widespread use of sulfa antibiotics, gamma globulin, and steroid drugs, facilitated the rapid growth of the NIH. Within two years, its budget grew to $4 million, and by 1950 it was up to $46.3 million. In 1948 another institute was added, the National Heart Institute, and the NIH became the National Institutes of Health. Its growth continued with the addition of several other new member institutes over the next twenty years. The focus of the NIH gradually shifted to "extramural" research—work conducted at the country's medical schools, hospitals, and universities rather than on the NIH campus itself.[2]

Thanks to the financial support of the NIH, subspecialty medical fellowships burgeoned during the postwar period. These fellowships paid for young doctors who had completed medical school, internship, and residency, to obtain additional clinical training in an area such as cardiology or nephrology or endocrinology and, most important, to develop research expertise in their chosen field. As a result of the largesse of the NIH, medicine moved from the province of the generalist to that of the specialist, and medical research metamorphosed from the pursuit of a privileged minority to a prestigious career, sought after by large numbers of the best and brightest physicians.[3] The most successful subspecialties were those that succeeded in carving out their own institutes within the NIH.

The prime movers behind the National Cancer Institute and the National Heart Institute, the earliest of the bunch, were two philanthropists, Florence Mahoney and Mary Lasker. Armed with their husbands' money—Mrs. Mahoney's husband owned the Cox newspapers and Mrs. Lasker's husband had made his millions in advertising—they developed a private, lay lobby for health research. They recognized that the best way to persuade congressmen to vote for new expenditures and to attract the public to their cause was to espouse a specific *disease*. The image of a hardworking family man struck down in his prime by a heart attack conjured up dread and sympathy in Congress, which was made up principally of middle-aged men. Real people suffering from real diseases were very difficult for legislators to ignore. This was evident when a man with kidney failure was wheeled onto the Senate floor to appeal for federal coverage of the full costs of dialysis. As a result, end-stage renal disease has been tacked on to Social Security as a special benefit.[4]

Researchers in the field of aging took to heart the lessons learned from the tremendous success of specialized institutes within the NIH and of the "categorical" (i.e., disease-specific) approach. Their first task was to establish a subdivision on aging, and the second was to target a single disease that afflicts the elderly. Many supporters of medical research failed to see any virtue in an institute dedicated to a phenomenon (aging), rather than an organ system (such as the heart or brain). Mary Lasker, for instance, remained skeptical. From her point of view, the major maladies of the elderly were heart disease and cancer. Their eradication—and she felt confident that their respective institutes would lead to their eradication—would "solve" the problem of aging. Her fellow philanthropist Florence Mahoney, however, made a sizable financial contribution. Congress came up with a matching gift and officially created the National Institute on Aging in 1975, devoted to "biomedical, social, and behavioral research on aging."

The NIA's first director, the psychiatrist Robert Butler, was convinced that the new institute needed a single disease as a focus. Citing the "politics of anguish," he said that only a disease with powerful emotional overtones could galvanize sufficient interest to make the NIA a success. Alzheimer's disease was the ideal choice. Butler also recognized the importance of winning over other specialists who might see Alzheimer's as their turf. The psychiatrists in the National Institute of Mental Health (NIMH), for instance, were inclined to regard Alzheimer's, with its effects on mood and behavior, as one of "their" diseases. The neurologists at the National Institute of Neurological and Communicative Disorders and Stroke (NINCDS) tended to see Alzheimer's as a brain disease and hence as "belonging" to them. Through clever diplomacy, Butler managed to persuade his counterparts at these two other institutes to support the NIA and to collaborate in the area of Alzheimer's disease.

The decision to make Alzheimer's disease its number one research priority was a tactical coup in the competition for federal dollars. It meshed beautifully with the prevailing ascendancy of "hard" science over social science: the public and their Congressmen believed in the primacy of health and in the ability of the medical profession to maintain health. Assuring other crucial components of a good quality of life in old age—adequate housing, access to personal care services, and above all retaining a sense of purpose—required messy social science research and were, in principle, far more difficult to achieve. The attention paid by the research establishment to Alzheimer's also fit in with the superior status of laboratory research relative to clinical research.[5] Scientists studying the underpinnings of Alzheimer's do their work at the bench, not at the bedside. They make their measurements on protein gels and centrifuges, not directly on people. The most prestigious work in the field of medicine is this kind of "basic science."

For headway to be made in tackling Alzheimer's disease, it was not enough to persuade researchers that the scientific puzzle was interesting, nor was it sufficient to persuade Congress that the science was worth funding; it was also imperative that the public become aware of the magnitude of the problem. Only if America as a whole believed in the crusade against dementia could individual citizens be relied on to provide private donations that complemented the federal handouts; only then could the voters be expected to demand the community services and other public programs that are the backbone of daily care for people with Alzheimer's.

The American people were won over to the cause of Alzheimer's disease by yet another critical player in the political process—the lay advocacy movement. The very same people who declared Alzheimer's to be a public health catastrophe and made it the centerpiece of the NIA—Robert Katzman and Robert Butler, respectively—also pushed for the establishment of a national lay organization devoted to

Alzheimer's. After an unsuccessful attempt at setting up an advocacy group in New York in1974, Robert Katzman tried again in 1978. This time, Katzman, whose mother-in-law had Alzheimer's, joined forces with Lonie Wollin, a New York attorney, three of whose family members had died of Alzheimer's, and with Jerome Stone, a Chicago businessman whose wife had Alzheimer's. They built an organization dedicated to public education, caregiver support, and the facilitation of research, primarily via lobbying efforts rather than direct grants.

The desire for advocacy groups was in the air, and miscellaneous other groups with similar goals began assembling in different states. Butler called all these lay groups to Washington, D.C., in 1979 in the hope that they would iron out their differences and form a single, united organization. Two months later, in December 1979, ADRDA (the Alzheimer's Disease and Related Disorders Association) held its first board meeting, electing Jerome Stone to the presidency.

The early success of ADRDA was due both to chance and to good organization. In its first year of existence, ADRDA stumbled upon a major publicity opportunity. The nationally syndicated newspaper column "Dear Abby" published a letter lamenting the difficulties of dealing with a demented relative. The column offered the name and address of ADRDA as a resource for others with similar concerns. Over the next few weeks, the fledgling organization received upwards of twenty-five-thousand requests for information.[6] The office rose to the occasion, assembling pamphlets, letters, and ultimately a book on Alzheimer's for the general public. The book started out as a few hand-mimeographed chapters that were put together and privately distributed at the suggestion of ADRDA by Nancy Mace and Peter Rabins of Johns Hopkins University. When the authors found themselves selling two-hundred copies a week of their homemade book, they decided to seek a publisher. One trade press after another turned them down, arguing that a book on Alzheimer's was too depressing and therefore unmarketable. Ultimately, Johns Hopkins University Press agreed to bring out the book with the title *The 36-Hour Day*. Now in its second edition, over half a million copies have been sold, making it one of the few bestsellers released by a university press. The book finally became available through a commercial press as well (Warners) in 1984 after it continued to sell between two thousand and three thousand copies a month.

The leadership of ADRDA saw their job as collaborating with scientists and policy makers, not merely fund-raising for them. As a result, ADRDA was the prime mover behind the hearings held by the Subcommittees on Aging of the House and the Senate. These hearings were a forum for experts of various kinds, members of assorted lobbying organizations for the aged such as the Gray Panthers and the American Association for Retired Persons (AARP), and caregivers for the demented elderly to get together to discuss perceptions, facts, and needs. In May 1983, the Senate Subcommittee on Aging held hearings on the "oversight and treatment" of Alzheimer's, which culminated in a document entitled "Endless Night, Endless Mourning: Living with Alzheimer's." A few days later, the House Select Committee on Aging held another hearing, also resulting in a publication, this one with the alliterative title "Senility, the Last Stereotype."

When formal criteria for diagnosing Alzheimer's disease were finally draw up and published in 1984, the individuals involved were representatives of the NIH and of ADRDA.[7] This document marked the end of an era in the history of Alzheimer's disease—the era in which "presenile" and "senile" dementia were regarded, though somewhat ambivalently, as distinct entities. It was also of symbolic significance, signaling Alzheimer's debut in the political arena. Alzheimer's disease was supported by a research institute of the NIH and by a mature lay advocacy organization. It was truly a national concern.

A Perpetual Political Battle

The establishment of the NIA, with Alzheimer's its centerpiece, and the birth of the lay advocacy movement were just the first of many political battles surrounding Alzheimer's. A sustained effort was critical to guarantee ongoing federal grant support for Alzheimer's research, and to maintain public awareness and interest.

At the federal level, politics influences the type and

amount of research done on Alzheimer's disease. Although all research proposals submitted to the NIH undergo rigorous peer review, much of the research on Alzheimer's disease is conducted by the Alzheimer's Disease Research Centers, which are subject to a special review process. In 1984, the NIH supported five centers; over the years these mushroomed to twenty-eight. Together they receive the lion's share of federal funding for biomedical research in Alzheimer's, which in turn represents about two thirds of the entire NIA budget.[8] Decisions about which hospitals or medical centers should be awarded the distinction of being an Alzheimer's Disease Research Center is in part a political one. Some centers have been far more productive and innovative than others, but are protected by a process that takes into consideration factors other than pure scientific merit.

The NIH also has an effect on what research is done through the allocation of funds among the various institutes—heart, cancer, aging, and so forth. Prevailing trends within the federal science bureaucracy as a whole influence the kind of science that is apt to be favorably regarded by the NIA. For instance, since 1991, a sizable chunk of NIH funds have gone to the Human Genome Project. This ambitious endeavor involves creating genetic maps of all twenty-three human chromosomes: finding "markers" on each region of every chromosome that can be used in locating specific genes. The next step is to find genes of interest in the area of each marker. The ultimate goal is to sequence all these genes, identifying the exact ordering of their base pairs (the genetic alphabet that spells out the protein composition of all DNA).[9] The extensive politicking that led to the adoption of the Human Genome Project by the NIH involved selling key people on the importance of finding genes related in some way to disease. Once this basic principle was accepted, any disease with a genetic component achieved special consideration. In the case of Alzheimer's disease, this meant plummeting into the spotlight the rare familial forms of the disease. As a result, many of the major recent advances in Alzheimer's research have involved the approximately 125 extended families worldwide who harbor a gene that invariably produces Alzheimer's disease.[10]

The belief that the discovery of the genetic basis of a rare form of Alzheimer's disease, accounting for at most 10 to 15 percent of all cases, would shed light on the pathogenesis of the other 85 to 90 percent fit in with the prevailing view that genetic information will provide the key to much if not most of human disease. The possibility of such a link was plausible, and the molecular basis of familial Alzheimer's disease is intriguing in its own right. But there is a compelling argument that the two, while related, are very different diseases. After all, pneumonia can be caused by bacteria or by viruses, and the clinical symptoms are very similar regardless of which kind of organism causes the mischief. Moreover, the pathogenesis—the way in which the microbes get into the lungs and then wreak their damage—is very similar. Both kinds of pneumonia are diagnosed by taking the patient's history, by listening to the lungs, and by a chest X ray. But the treatment for bacterial pneumonia is antibiotics, while the only available treatment for viral pneumonia is "tincture of time." Antibiotics are generally useless for viral pneumonia.

Another example of a similar phenomenon is the two different types of angina (chest pain due to insufficient oxygen to the heart). The more common cause of angina is blockage of the coronary arteries, the vessels carrying oxygen and other nutrients to the heart muscle. The blockage is usually caused by atherosclerosis, by debris building up on the walls of the coronary arteries as a result of damage to the vessel lining from longstanding high blood pressure or elevated cholesterol. There is, however, a second much less common form of angina that causes the same kind of chest pain but that is due to spasm of the coronary arteries. This variety, called Prinzmetal's angina, cannot be treated with coronary artery bypass surgery or the Roto-Rooter treatment known as angioplasty. Some medications are effective in both kinds of angina, but others work in one and not the other.

Many prominent researchers are convinced that once they identify the protein coded for by the newly discovered genes, and once the role of that protein in normal bodily processes is identified, they will have all the clues needed to put together a model of Alzheimer's disease. As Nobel Prize winner James Watson put it: "Are we going to find out what Alzheimer's is and why it causes brain failure without getting the genes that we know predispose certain people to the disease? Maybe we will, but I would not bet on it. But if we can get the gene or genes implicated in the disease, I am confident that we will save hundreds of millions of dollars, if not billions, that would have been spent on worthless research."[11] Blueprint of the disease in hand, they will be ready for a frontal assault. This conviction is more a reflection of ideology than of reality. It is rooted in the belief that genetic information will go a long way toward explaining many if not most diseases, which is the underlying premise of the Human Genome Project. The conviction that knowledge about genes will produce cures for human disease has influenced fields as disparate as cardiology and oncology. It is not surprising that the study of Alzheimer's, some variants of which clearly do have a genetic basis, should be powerfully influenced by the dominant ideology.

The Congress has been generous in its support of Alzheimer's disease over the past fifteen years. It has repeatedly allocated special funds for Alzheimer's, outside the unwieldy NIH budget process. For example, it created an Alzheimer's Disease Education Center in 1986 and then in 1989 appropriated an extra $20 million for Alzheimer's disease on a special, onetime basis. This support, however, is at the whim of legislators. In an era in which Congress is trying desperately to balance the budget and articles appear in the media decrying the "excessive" expenditures on the elderly, "soft money" (that is, grants) that underlie much of the American research effort could easily vanish.[12] Zaven Khachaturian, for many years the head of the neurosciences section of the NIA and a forceful spokesperson for Alzheimer's disease research, has left the federal government to head the new private Reagan Research Institute. The current director of the NIA, Richard Hodes, is himself a basic scientist and is widely expected to move the organization in the direction of greater commitment to molecular biology rather than specific diseases such as Alzheimer's. Scientific advances in the field of Alzheimer's disease (which are far from guaranteed to produce a cure but which are our only hope for finding any effective treatment) do not occur spontaneously. They depend on a highly political funding process—a mechanism whose wheels require extensive greasing, and whose spark plugs need frequent replacement for the engine to keep on running.[13]

Just as federal funding for Alzheimer's research can never be considered secure, neither can public support be taken for granted. Since its formation, the Alzheimer's Disease and Related Disorders Association (ADRDA), recently renamed the Alzheimer's Association, has participated in diverse aspects of the politics of Alzheimer's disease. One of the association's many highly successful strategies is to disseminate human interest stories in the news media and in its own publications. These stories serve to educate the public about Alzheimer's, to provide comfort to caregivers, who often identify strongly with the plight of the families described, and to elicit contributions by playing on readers' fears and anxieties. The Alzheimer's Association also does the usual things that advocacy groups do: it hires lobbyists to work in Congress, it creates support groups, and it prints glossy brochures about various aspects of the disease. The organization has grown enormously: by 1986, it had 125 chapters with affiliates in forty-four states. As of 1995, it was composed of a network of over 220 local chapters, 2,000 support groups, and 35,000 volunteers.

Underlying the organizational strategy of the Alzheimer's Association is a single unifying theme: dementia is distinct from normal aging. Over and over, the association's literature and spokesmen at conferences hammer home this point. They do so partly to counteract the widespread belief that "senility" is a normal concomitant of aging—more common at the time of the organization's inception, but still prevalent today. They also stress that dementia is a disease—convinced that only if dementia is regarded as a medical problem will it garner any public support.[14] If dementia in general and Alzheimer's in particular are medical problems, then they warrant funding of scientific research aimed toward cure. If dementia is a disease rather than an inevitable part of aging, then afflicted individuals should be treated in "adult day health centers" in the community and "special care units" within nursing homes, just as cardiac patients are cared for in coronary care units.

The conscious decision to emphasize the biomedical aspects of Alzheimer's disease, while very successful in achieving its objectives, has furthered the already pervasive trend toward the "medicalization" of aging. Framing dementia as principally a medical problem lends credence to the view that the problems of aging are primarily due to physiological decline: "The phenomenon and experience of aging are brought within the medical paradigm as individual pathology to be treated and cured."[15] A competing view is that there are at least as many nonmedical issues—such as poverty, isolation, and the loss of role and status—that contribute to the problems of aging. From this perspective, designating Alzheimer's as a disease in order to promote acceptability and fundability is just as suspect as defining alcoholism as a disease or, in the not so distant past, labeling homosexuality as abnormal.

The Alzheimer's movement may well have gone too far in its insistence on distinguishing Alzheimer's from aging. Interestingly, scientists themselves are questioning the disease model they have endorsed for the last twenty years. Allen Roses of Duke University stated that "what is called Alzheimer's disease may not be a 'disease' at all, but a natural part of the aging process."[16] A recent conference put together by the prestigious medical journal *Lancet* asked but did not answer the question: "Is cognitive deterioration a continuous age-related process or is it a discrete disease pathology?"[17] At the very least, many researchers suggest redefining Alzheimer's as a syndrome (a cluster of symptoms) that may have multiple distinct etiologies.[18] This view is generated in part by new scientific discoveries, in part by epidemiologic data, and in part by the *political* realization that we do not need to classify Alzheimer's as a disease to justify attempts to ameliorate its symptoms. On the contrary, if dementia is the ultimate fate for most of us, we are more obligated than ever to figure out how to stave it off as long as possible and, once we get it, how to live with it.

Keeping Alzheimer's disease and normal aging separate in the public eye may no longer be necessary to garner support for research, but there is no doubt that it was a very successful strategy. Some commentators suggest that the approaches used by the Alzheimer's movement have been *too* successful—they have led to the "alzheimerization" of gerontologic research. Many other aspects of aging do not receive nearly as much attention (measured principally in research dollars) as Alzheimer's disease; much more government spending goes to the "applied" field of Alzheimer's disease research than to "basic" studies of the process of aging.[19] The advocacy movement intended to promote the welfare of those with Alzheimer's and their caregivers accomplished a great deal. Without resorting to the confrontational tactics of other lay groups and without relegating itself to a minor role in a field dominated by professional scientists and physicians, the Alzheimer's Association has made a difference in how Sylvia Truman and her family, and others like them, experience dementia.

Politics and New Drugs: The Tacrine Story

When an article was published in a major medical journal in 1986 proclaiming the efficacy of a new drug in the treatment of Alzheimer's disease, I thought there had been a remarkable breakthrough. The study, although small (only seventeen people enrolled and only fourteen entered the final phase), reported that one subject was able to resume part-time work, one returned to his golf game, and another went back to homemaking. Quantitative tests of cognitive function and global rating scales—an overall assessment of the participants' functioning in daily life—both revealed statistically significant improvement in the treated group. The lead author of the study cautioned that the new medication was no more a cure for Alzheimer's than Sinemet was for Parkinson's—but Sinemet, while assuredly not a cure for Parkinson's, has dramatically ameliorated the stiffness and slowness associated with Parkinson's. If the new medicine for Alzheimer's disease was remotely like the medicine for Parkinson's, it was indeed a marvel.[20]

The drug was known by the inauspicious name tetrahydroaminoacridine, or, more familiarly, tacrine. The rationale for its use was analogous to the rationale for Sinemet: just as the brains of Parkinson's patients lack the neurochemical dopamine, so the brains of Alzheimer's patients are strikingly deficient in another neurotransmitter, acetylcholine. Just as Sinemet is a replacement for the missing chemical, so, too, tacrine was intended to boost the corresponding chemical that is missing with Alzheimer's. Tacrine works through an indirect mechanism: it inhibits the action of a naturally occurring substance whose job is to destroy acetylcholine. By this double-negative approach, tacrine augments brain levels of acetylcholine.

The role of acetylcholine in memory and of its absence in Alzheimer's had been known since work in the early 1970s linking acetylcholine and memory, and subsequent studies showing that patients with Alzheimer's disease had a marked decrease in acetylcholine-dependent neurons (see Chapter 2). Seemingly all that was needed was biochemical tinkering and, eventually, a suitable molecule would be found to treat Alzheimer's effectively. The study of tacrine appeared to herald the arrival of just such a drug.

An editorial accompanying the article praised the strategy as a "triumph for the scientific method."[21] The news media immediately picked up on the study, and the Alzheimer's Association was bombarded with requests for information on how to procure the new drug. William Summers, the lead author of the study, filed an application for a new investigational drug with the Food and Drug Administration (FDA), the federal organization empowered to evaluate whether new drugs were sufficiently safe and effective to be marketed. Science, the pharmaceutical industry, and the government regulatory system were all working together to produce a cure for a dread disease.

Or so it seemed. But something was amiss. There were rumblings within the scientific community. Who was William Summers? He was a psychiatrist at the UCLA School of Medicine who had been interested for some time in acetylcholine and its cousins as a means of treating Alzheimer's disease. A small-circulation journal, *Biological Psychiatry,* published a preliminary study by Summers and his collaborators in 1981.[22] Otherwise, he had published a total of fifteen articles (excluding letters to the editor) prior to 1986, all but one in psychiatric journals and minor general medical journals. Except for two tacrine articles (the pilot study mentioned and one review article), the papers reported on small studies of assorted psychiatric topics, including shock treatment and manic-depressive disorder. Whoever he was, the department in which he worked was not one of the major sites for Alzheimer's research.

Not all the criticism revolved around Summers himself. Neurologists wondered about Summers's methodology. Were all the patients carefully evaluated to be sure that they really did have Alzheimer's disease—as sure as is possible, short of a brain biopsy? Were the outcome measures—the scales of cognitive function and the "global assessment ratings"—truly meaningful? Individuals treated with tacrine performed better on these various tests than those not given tacrine, and the differences were statistically significant, but did they translate into changes of any real-life consequence? And wasn't it a bit premature to jump to conclusions based on a study conducted on only seventeen people?

The Summers paper was tantalizing. But only a large-scale trial, a study involving hundreds of patients and thus necessitating the cooperation of investigators at many clinical sites, all of whom adhered to rigorous criteria drawn up in advance for eligibility and who followed the same clearly specified protocol, could answer the question of whether tacrine was useful for Alzheimer's. The National Institute on Aging, the National Institutes of Health, and the Alzheimer's Association agreed to sponsor such an ambitious study jointly, and the Tacrine Collaborative Study Group was born.

Before the collaborative completed its work, tacrine made the headlines again. This time it was in the form of a frontal attack by the Food and Drug Administration (FDA), which came just short of accusing Summers of fraud. The agency, in an unusual "interim report" published in the *New England Journal*, the same journal that had printed Summers's earlier results, acknowledged that it had not uncovered any "clear evidence of purposeful misrepresentation."[23] However, as soon as Summers had applied for tacrine to be an investigational drug, the FDA, as was its custom, had begun an inquiry into the research underlying his conclusions. The FDA was appalled to find little documentation that the study had actually been conducted as described in the journal article. The means by which patients were randomized were never clear, it was not certain whether the study physicians were in fact in

the dark about who was on tacrine and who was taking placebo during the trial, and the "global" assessments were either
recorded in a very sloppy fashion or were decided upon *after*
completion of the study. All these procedural issues, plus puz-
zlement as to how Summers had managed to remain unaware
of the strong tendency for tacrine to cause liver toxicity, led
the FDA to conclude that Summers's work constituted no
more than anecdotal data. Moreover, officials at the FDA
were clearly very angry: an irate public vilified them as heart-
lessly impeding the relief of suffering and demanded the
immediate release of tacrine. David Kessler, head of the FDA,
reported receiving hate mail from writers asserting that "the
time is long past for being polite and courteous and willing to
wait while the FDA wastes the lives of five million victims."
Feeling that the work that had precipitated such animosity
was deeply flawed, the scientists at the FDA could barely contain their antagonism. The study, by virtue of its prominent
publication, had set in motion "premature request for wide
distribution of the drug . . . [and] caused those who care for
the victims of Alzheimer's disease needless anguish, leading
them to believe that their loved ones were being denied
access to a drug of established efficacy and value."[24]

The FDA's comments bring into relief the conflicting
views of the activist public—which wants any new drug that
appears promising to be made immediately available—and
the regulatory agency, which seeks to protect the populace
from seemingly good drugs that might prove to be dangerous
or ineffective. They also demonstrate the dramatic conflict
between the political arena, in which the horizon for change
is no longer than the next election, and the scientific arena,
in which progress requires years of fastidious work. Despite
the lack of success of the "War on Cancer" (declared by
Richard Nixon in 1971, with no armistice in sight as of 1997),
the public tends to equate successful science with other large,
federally run endeavors such as the Manhattan Project or the
space mission. The Manhattan Project gave massive government support to a whole enclave of scientists and technicians
who, over a period of three years, developed an atomic bomb.
Similarly, though on a smaller scale, the pressures of World
War II impelled the federal government to fund the development of penicillin. The military recognized that many soldiers

who died were felled by virulent microbes that infested battle wounds rather than by enemy fire. Aware that a new drug existed with remarkable antibacterial properties, the federal government set in motion a large-scale research effort to bring penicillin to the battlefield.

Applying existing technology to a challenging problem is a very different matter from uncovering the mechanism of a disease. In the case of penicillin, the problem was not establishing that bacteria caused disease (Robert Koch had done so in the 1880s) or finding a substance that could kill germs without killing their human hosts (Alexander Fleming had done that in 1928 when he discovered penicillin); all that was needed was to determine which of the numerous types of disease-causing bacteria were destroyed by penicillin, how much of the drug to give, and how to obtain large quantities in a short period at a reasonable cost. In the case of Alzheimer's disease, where the factors causing and facilitating the development of the disorder remain obscure, the prospects for finding a treatment by declaring war are extremely remote.

The next chapter in the tacrine story was the publication of the eagerly awaited study by the Tacrine Collaborative Study Group in 1992. The results indicated that tacrine *did* have a measurable effect in people with mild to moderate Alzheimer's. The authors concluded that "treatment resulted in a statistically significant reduction in decline of cognitive function, although this reduction was not large enough to be detected by the study physicians' global assessments of the patients."[25] A vindication of Summers's work? In an accompanying editorial, the neurologist and prominent researcher John Growdon argued that the differences between the tacrine Group and the controls were "clinically trivial." Given the minimal efficacy of tacrine together with its increasingly evident liver toxicity, Growdon was skeptical about its usefulness.[26]

The story was not over. On September 9, 1993, in what seemed to be an about-face, the FDA approved tacrine for use in Alzheimer's disease. Its decision was determined in large part by the results of yet another study, soon to be published in the *Journal of the American Medical Association*. This paper looked at the effect of a higher dose of tacrine (double the dose used previously) given for a longer period of time (thirty weeks instead of six or twelve). The patients who tolerated the highest dose demonstrated statistically *and clinically* observed improvements on objective tests *and global evaluations* by both physicians and caregivers. The verdict, it seemed, was in.[27]

A closer look at this seemingly definitive study raised new concerns. Two of the authors, including the lead author, were paid employees of the Warner-Lambert Company, the manufacturer of tacrine. Not only were they salaried by Warner-Lambert, but they also owned stock and stock options in the company. Clearly their work is not *invalidated* by their drug company connection, but many regard it as tarnished because they have a financial interest in tacrine's becoming a bestselling medication. Researchers always stand to gain personally if their investigations are successful: they gain in prestige and in promotions. But the possibility of pecuniary gain raises the stakes to new levels. Even the appearance of conflict of interest may hopelessly taint drug company–sponsored research in the eyes of the clinicians and other scientists who evaluate its credibility.

Apart from the credentials of the investigators, the new findings presented another problem. Fully 70 percent of the subjects enrolled in the highest dose group, the one group to demonstrate considerable improvement, dropped out of the study. They dropped out either because of abnormal liver function tests induced by the medication or because of intolerable gastrointestinal side effects (nausea and vomiting). The extraordinarily high attrition rate called into question the advisability of even trying a drug that most patients could not take.

Tacrine is on the market now, sold under the brand name of Cognex. A second, similar drug is also now available, donepezil (Aricept). This medication works the same way as tacrine but without any reports of liver toxicity, though it causes the same gastrointestinal side effects. It is also easier to take since it is a once-a-day medication. There is only one published study of its efficacy, though two other unpublished studies (neither of which compares donepezil to tacrine) apparently show the same modest improvements as with tacrine. Based on these limited studies, the FDA approved donepezil in November 1996.

Why should a single medication generate such strong emotions? Does the controversy truly arise from a desire to protect patients from having their hopes dashed by a drug that promises more than it delivers? Is the issue really toxicity, given that the dangers involved are quite small and are readily reversible by discontinuing the medication? Surely the furor engendered by tacrine has been disproportionate to either its risks or its benefits. The basis for the hoopla has had at least as much to do with politics as with tacrine.

The Medical-Industrial Complex

The corporate world played a role in the tacrine controversy, with Warner-Lambert, the manufacturer of the drug, subsidizing much of the research on its efficacy. Other companies are players in the political arena as well, influencing what questions are asked and which answers are publicized. No longer is sophisticated science the exclusive province of academic departments at major universities; a bevy of firms have sprung up that are devoted to science but have the additional goal of producing marketable products rather than research papers. Sporting names such as Athena Neurosciences (an allusion to the Greek goddess of wisdom) and Cephalon (meaning pertaining to the head), these companies play a growing role in scientific development. At a recent molecular biology meeting, 25 percent of all papers presented came from the corporate sector.[28]

For-profit, private firms have quietly insinuated themselves into the business of laboratory science for some time. The public first learned of the phenomenon when the Nobel Prize–winning biologist Walter Gilbert resigned his professorship at Harvard to become chief executive officer of a biotechnology company, Biogen. He believed that venture capital and ultimately the public, in the form of shareholders, would fund scientific endeavors on a far more generous scale than would the NIH, which was increasingly afflicted by budget cutbacks. As molecular biology became progressively mechanized, Gilbert recognized that genetically engineered antibodies or even synthetic genes could be created in large enough quantities to be commercially useful. Two years later, with Biogen doing poorly, Gilbert returned to Harvard as chairman of the Biology Department. But the temptation to join—and shape—the world of industry remained strong, and in 1987 Gilbert started yet another biotech firm.

Alzheimer's disease research, like many other branches of medicine, has been dramatically affected by the growth of start-up companies. Not surprisingly, private industry views Alzheimer's as a potential growth area since the disorder affects 2.5 million people in the United States and perhaps as many as 22 million worldwide. Of great commercial interest would be a diagnostic test that could be used to determine who among the even larger population of individuals with some degree of memory impairment actually have Alzheimer's. A second kind of highly profitable test would be a predictive test. Anyone who is at risk for the disease by virtue of age or family history, even if he or she currently has no symptoms, might be sufficiently apprehensive about developing Alzheimer's in the future to be persuaded to undergo such a test. A treatment for Alzheimer's—a cure for those already affected—would of course be a fantastic boon for those with the disease and for the pharmaceutical company that patented the drug.

Companies have seized upon all three of these avenues of investigation. In the diagnostic realm, one of the leads pursued was a skin biopsy. Dennis Selkoe, a prominent researcher working on the structure and function of amyloid, reported in 1989 that he had found antibodies against amyloid in tissues other than the brain, including skin.[29] This finding was of interest from a theoretical point of view because it suggested that Alzheimer's might be a systemic disease rather than a localized brain disease: the neuron-destroying amyloid might arrive in the brain via the bloodstream rather than arising from defective handling of amyloid precursor protein inside the brain itself. From a practical point of view, it was tremendously exciting: the demonstration of anti-amyloid antibodies in the skin, if found uniquely in patients with Alzheimer's, could potentially lead to a cheap, safe, and easy diagnostic test. A skin biopsy, unlike a brain biopsy, currently the only definitive diagnostic test for Alzheimer's during life, is associated with virtually no risk. The drug company Bristol-Myers Squibb, tantalized by the possibility of an easy test for Alzheimer's, awarded Selkoe a $500,000 grant to study the phenomenon further and hopefully develop a reliable test. Selkoe's group had been exploring far more fundamental questions related to how Alzheimer's disease developed; a foray into the arena of diagnostic testing, while potentially extremely valuable, constituted a diversion from Selkoe's main research program. As it turned out, the test proved unreliable and was abandoned.

Another possible diagnostic test that got extensive media publicity is the eyedrop test. This test involves putting a few drops in the eye and carefully measuring how much the pupil dilates. In people with Alzheimer's disease, early studies showed a marked increase in response compared to normal controls. The test is still under study, but so far it is not sufficiently accurate to be used in everyday clinical practice.[30]

New tests that purport to simplify the diagnosis of Alzheimer's disease continue to emerge, such as the AD7C test marketed by the Nymox Corporation, which measures the level of a protein known as 21kD NTP in the spinal fluid. Nymox claims in its promotional literature that it is "the first test proven to help physicians be certain in the diagnosis of Alzheimer's disease." The director of the Alzheimer Disease Research Centers Program at the NIA commented in response that "a recurring theme for most new Alzheimer's disease diagnostics is that they tend to get marketed and hyped before the data are available in large populations." AD7C is no different—its alleged usefulness is based on unpublished studies showing that it allows doctors to distinguish between patients with Alzheimer's disease and people without dementia, a feat they should be able to perform with a clinical examination. Nymox charges $1000 for the test, which does not include the cost of the spinal tap necessary to obtain the fluid for analysis.[31]

A reliable predictive test for Alzheimer's disease could be targeted to a huge market. All individuals worried about developing the disease at some point in the future are potential candidates for such a test. Identifying in advance who is destined to develop a serious illness is useful if it has consequences for the person's decisions about having children or if early diagnosis can lead to early treatment. Screening for carriers of Tay-Sachs disease, for example, a condition in which babies fail to develop normally and invariably die by about age two, has clear reproductive implications: a couple, both of whom carry one copy of the Tay-Sachs gene and thus have a one out of four chance of having an affected child, might choose not to have children, to adopt, or to undergo amnio-centesis to diagnose the condition in the womb, with the plan to abort a fetus carrying the disease. Screening individuals for a gene predisposing to breast cancer might encourage high-risk women to seek regular mammograms, which in turn may lead to diagnosis at a time when cure is possible.[32] Alzheimer's disease, with its typical age of onset in the seventies or eighties, does not fit the model of a disease in which screening is clearly beneficial. Nonetheless, companies such as Athena Neurosciences, a San Francisco biotechnology company devoted entirely to neurology research, are marketing screening tests for Alzheimer's. Picking up on a lead from Allen Roses, chairman of the Department of Neurology at Duke University, a prominent scientist and a stockholder in Athena Neurosciences, the company bought out a firm that packaged screening kits for apolipoprotein E. The kits are being sold for use in individuals at risk for Alzheimer's.[33]

Pharmaceutical firms bring enormous resources to bear in the struggle to find a treatment for Alzheimer's. The patient's best interests and those of the drug company giants do not necessarily coincide, as the profit motive leads corporations to protect their investments, to sell a drug they have spent millions in developing. Warner-Lambert and its parent company, Parke-Davis, continue to promote Cognex (tacrine) despite its poor reputation. Parke-Davis subsidizes informa-tional pamphlets created and distributed by the Alzheimer's Association, but on the back of the brochure is a sticker exhorting patients: "Ask your doctor about a new treatment program for Alzheimer's disease." "Treatment program" is a euphemism for tacrine. Although most researchers currently believe that effective treatment for Alzheimer's will come from an approach other than neurotransmitter replacement therapy, new tacrinelike drugs continue to be developed such as donepezil. Drug companies are pursuing other avenues as well: the amyloid supporters are interested in ways to block the neuron-damaging effects of amyloid, or to prevent amyloid from being formed in the first place, and the tau supporters are also interested in neuronal protection strategies, as well as in drugs that might impede the production of the abnormal form of tau.

To facilitate the search for treatment, several for-profit laboratories have developed animal models of Alzheimer's. In addition to Athena Neurosciences, the Marion Merrell Dow Research Institute (a drug company spinoff) and Scios Nova, another biotech start-up, have succeeded in implanting a human gene for Alzheimer's into a mouse. These experimental animals develop pathological changes that are similar to those found in people, though whether they develop analogous behavioral changes remains uncertain. Interestingly, the most recent mouse model, which develops both amyloid plaques and memory deficits, was produced in academia and will be supplied to other academic researchers without restricting its use.[34]

On balance, is involvement by for-profit corporations in medical research a good thing? Traditionally, the university has been the site of basic research, which is then applied by industry to create marketable products. The university is characterized, in theory, by openness, by the free exchange of information; the motivation of academic scientists is knowledge for its own sake. The private corporation, by contrast, is characterized by secrecy and its motivation is making money. These nice clean distinctions broke down long ago, as industry began to fund more and more basic science—surpassing the NIH for the first time in 1982. By 1993, NIH spent $10 billion per year on biomedical research; private companies spent slightly more, with drug companies alone expending over $6 billion and employing more than thirty thousand workers in research and development.[35] Not only do for-profit companies extensively support relatively fundamental research, but scientists at universities increasingly hope to supplement their incomes and to have an impact on the larger world by doing applied research.

Anxiety persists as the boundaries blur between basic and applied research, but many of the concerns about the dangers of privatizing science have proved unfounded. In principle, academic scientists with industry connections might be expected to steer their graduate students in directions of interest to the company but not necessarily in the best interest of the students' careers. In theory, university-based scientists doing product-oriented work might be expected to shirk their teaching or administrative responsibilities, to publish less in peer-reviewed journals, and to patent more.[36] In fact, a study by the Office of Technology Assessment concluded that those scientists with major industrial agreements both published and taught more than their counterparts without such connections.[37]

The image of the universities as promoting openness and cooperation is often just as outdated as the image of the corporation as a fortress, deliberately inaccessible to the rest of the world. In the case of Alzheimer's research, the competition among academic groups is so fierce that they are sometimes as secretive as biotech firms. Writing in 1992, Daniel Pollen, a scientist who chronicled the search for the genetic component of Alzheimer's disease, commented that "accounts of one group refusing to share cell lines with another or providing only limited samples to colleagues continue to circulate." Writing after the discovery of a gene for Alzheimer's located on chromosome 14, Pollen adds: "At times, even the integrity of the race was threatened by ruthless assaults on accepted standards governing the conduct of competition in science." He notes that a grant application submitted to the NIH by two of the leading groups working on identifying the gene was summarily dismissed based on the comments of a single reviewer who was apparently from a competing group.[38]

Just as the boundary between academia and industry has become blurred, so too has the separation between public and private. In the past, NIH money went to scientists who were expected to foster the growth of scientific knowledge, who were situated either at universities or on the NIH campus in Maryland. Since 1980, the federal government's philosophy has changed. With the passage of the Bayh-Dole Act, private industry has been expected to reap a profit from government collaboration: the act allowed small businesses to patent inventions arising from federally funded research. Under the Reagan administration, the same right was accorded big business. Since the introduction of CRADAs (Cooperative

Research and Development Agreements), NIH employees are entitled to earn 15 percent of royalties on patents, up to $100,000 per year. The Technology Transfer Act of 1986 effectively told government employees that it was their "patriotic duty to collaborate with industry to speed publicly funded research getting to the public." In keeping with this directive, NINDS (National Institute of Neurological Disease and Stroke) scientist Craig Venter announced that he planned to partially sequence all the genes active in the brain and patent them. If all had gone according to plan, NIH would have filed for one thousand patents a month. Venter's proposal stimulated tremendous controversy both within the NIH and in the biotechnology world. Could human genes be patented? And even if they could be, what about random pieces of DNA whose protein product (if any) was unknown and whose biological function was equally mysterious? James Watson, director of the Human Genome Project and éminence grise of molecular biology, responded contemptuously that "virtually any monkey" with a sequencing machine could sequence random segments of DNA.[39] Venter's concern, however, was that if he did not patent the sequences and they later proved to be valuable, they would then be in the public domain, unpatentable, and therefore, no company would make them commercially available. Bernardine Healy, NIH director at the time, supported Venter, arguing that "the rationale [of the patents] is not to make money, but rather to promote and encourage the development and commercialization of products to benefit the public and to do so in a socially responsible way."[40] Ironically, the Industrial Biotechnology Association, a trade group representing 80 percent of U.S. biotech investments, issued a position paper urging that the NIH *not* seek patent protection of DNA sequences of unknown function.[41] Ultimately, the U.S. Patent Office rejected the application on the grounds that the gene fragments failed to meet any of the three criteria for patentability: nonobviousness, novelty, and utility. The office described the application as "vague, indefinite, misdescriptive, incomplete, inaccurate, and incomprehensible."[42]

Venter left his position at NIH to head the newly founded private Institute for Genomic Research. Bankrolled by a $70 million, ten-year agreement with a corporate partner, Human

Genome Sciences, Inc., the Institute carried on Venter's work with the help of fast, expensive equipment, including fifty DNA sequencing machines, several workstations, and a super-computer.[43] Underneath the politicking and hostility lay a fundamental question: of what value are patents? Do they promote research by protecting a company's investment in commercializing its discoveries? Do they foster productive relationships between academia and industry by allowing universities to patent their discoveries and then license them to commercial firms that can bring out a product? Or do patents simply generate huge legal costs—both for the application process and for suits defending patent rights—without producing any unequivocally positive results? The resolution of the debate is not yet clear, but the controversy over patents reveals the extent of the entanglement between the public and private sectors.

Whether or not linkages between the private and public arenas, the corporate world and the academic world constitute an improvement over the earlier era of separation, they represent a feature of the research terrain that is likely to be with us for the foreseeable future. And they prove conclusively that developments in the area of Alzheimer's are intimately bound up with all sorts of concerns outside the narrow questions of the cause and cure for dementia.

The political backdrop is a crucial part of the Alzheimer's disease landscape: from the decision of the NIA in the 1970s to concentrate on a single disease, Alzheimer's, in order to establish its reputation, to the congressional legislation in the 1980s promoting corporate biomedical research, to the approval of tacrine and then donepezil by the FDA in the 1990s. Not only is politics important in the narrowest sense—in terms of law and regulations and funding—but also in the larger sense of all those factors outside the realm of Alzheimer's disease research that have an impact on the field. The effectiveness of the Alzheimer's Association in publicity and education has had a profound effect on the number and type of programs and studies of Alzheimer's. Broader trends in the scientific community, such as the contemporary emphasis on molecular genetics, exert a powerful influence on the direction pursued by neuroscientists interested in dementia. Change in how we view Alzheimer's and how Sylvia Truman experiences it are as much the result of the pharmaceutical industry's profit-maximization goals and the growth of the medical-industrial complex as they are of scientific successes.

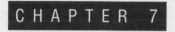

CHAPTER 7

Nightfall

The crisis the Truman family had been expecting was nearly a year in coming. They had suspected it was coming when they visited Sylvia in her apartment and detected an odor—not a very strong odor, not an entirely convincing odor, but a smell vaguely reminiscent of the subway stations in downtown Boston. "Did you smell something?" John asked his wife after they left. Cynthia had not been planning to mention anything. She didn't want to spoil their Mother's Day visit. But she knew immediately that John was not asking her whether the roses they had brought had a scent.

It was a faint smell that had struck them both the moment they came in. John commented that the apartment was stuffy—his mother, like many of her peers, kept the thermostat at eighty and had not turned the heat off even though it was May. He opened the windows, and after a few minutes the odor diffused away or the Trumans adapted to it. In any event, they ceased being aware of the distinctive and unpleasant odor of urine.

"I thought I did," Cynthia admitted. "But I didn't notice any wet spots or any stains on the carpet. I was a little afraid to sit down on the sofa, but the seats seemed okay."

"Maybe Mom's gotten herself a puppy." John laughed in my office when he acknowledged the lengths he had been willing to go to deny the obvious. "Or maybe one of her friends has a little problem."

Sylvia had found friends at the assisted living facility. They weren't the companions her family would have chosen for her, but at least Sylvia was not alone so much. Maxine wore red lipstick that she could not quite manage to confine to her lips, giving her mouth a boxy, horsey appearance. She used eyeshadow and blush, which accentuated rather than disguised her age. She went to the beauty parlor weekly, where she had her hair dyed, permed, and brushed into a small haystack configuration. Maxine wore large earrings, bright clothes, and heels that were dangerously high. She liked dance music from the thirties and frequently played samples from her scratched record collection for Sylvia. She went shopping with Sylvia in the van provided by the apartment complex, and both of them came back with shirts they did not need in colors that did not suit them. Jenny had had a below-the-knee amputation because of diabetes, and wore a prosthesis. She used a walker and was in and out of the hospital for heart problems and infections in her remaining foot. She talked incessantly, telling the same stories repeatedly, with minor variations. Her stories were about her four children, none of whom Sylvia had ever met because they never came to see their mother. She talked about her dog, who had been dead for thirty years, and the parakeet she had been forced to relinquish when she moved into the assisted living building. The real reason that the Truman family could not abide Maxine and Jenny was that they found their cognitive impairment painful to witness. They resembled Sylvia in their limitations, but Sylvia they could love for who she had been. They could treasure what remained of her stubbornness and her generosity; Maxine and Jenny seemed to them caricatures of their former selves.

"I think Jenny was hospitalized with a bladder infection," Cynthia volunteered. "I've heard that sometimes infections can cause incontinence." She had finally said the word aloud.

"Or maybe it was Mom," John remarked.

They decided to drop the subject, to wait and see if they noticed anything on their next visit. John went over weekly to pay his mother's bills and to bring her any supplies she needed.

The following week the weather was mild and the windows were wide open. The apartment was clean—once a week a

housekeeper vacuumed and dusted and did the laundry—
and if it smelled at all, it was the faint aroma of lemon furniture polish. But John was surprised to find that there were no
sheets on the bed.

"Doesn't the housekeeper change your linens, Mom?"
John asked, puzzled.

"Yes," Sylvia responded tersely. She tended not to provide
any more information than absolutely necessary, partly because she had difficulty finding the words to express herself,
partly because she had become more concrete in her
thinking and interpreted questions literally, unable to detect
implicit queries.

"So didn't she change your sheets this week?"

"She did. But I had to take them off."

"What happened, Mom?"

"They got wet."

"Did you have an accident?"

"No, I didn't have an accident." To Sylvia, an accident
meant falling, like the time she had broken her hip. "It
happened while I was sleeping." Accidents, evidently, only
occurred to people who were up and about.

"A wet dream," John joked, but Sylvia did not grasp the joke.

"It just came out." John could see that his mother was
embarrassed, and he stopped trying to tease her. He ex-
tracted the details from her, as best as she could recall them:
she had woken up soaked; she had put the sheets in a garbage
bag and shoved it in the back of the closet; she could not
figure out how to make the bed with fresh linen and the
housekeeper was not due for a few more days—she wasn't
sure whether she came on Tuesdays or Wednesdays. Apparently she had never wet the bed before, and she denied
having any problems during the day.

John wasn't sure what to do. The memories of his Mother's
Day suspicions wafted back to him, but he repressed them.
He was certain of only one episode; he would wait to see if
this event was an isolated occurrence or part of a pattern.

When the director of the assisted living facility called John
and Marcia for an urgent family meeting, John concluded
that the incontinence had not been a onetime accident
and that the crisis he had been anticipating had arrived. The

director was gentle but firm. Sylvia was leaving puddles on chairs in the common areas; her dresses were stained; her apartment smelled. She delivered an ultimatum: something had to be done, or Sylvia's lease, which was due for renewal in another month, would be terminated. She was cautiously optimistic. Incontinence was a common problem in the elderly with dementia, but in many cases it could be cured or at least ameliorated.[1] She would like to keep Sylvia in the facility—she was a lovely lady, forgetful and frequently disoriented, but polite and quiet—but all the other tenants were talking about her. Maxine tried to cover up for her and clean up after her. Jenny, who was unsteady on her feet and could not make beds or do laundry, had given her a bottle of perfume and a large can of aerosol deodorant. Apparently Sylvia's trouble had started some months earlier, but her leaking had been rare and her friends had successfully shielded her from notice.

John and Marcia were touched by the devotion of Sylvia's much maligned friends, and they were terrified by the director's demand. What if Sylvia's incontinence could not be fixed? Would she need to enter a nursing home? How could they find a good place for her in a month? What if she had to stay with them for a while? Would they have to drape the upholstery with plastic covers? Should they buy adult diapers for Sylvia?

A week later, the three of them were in my office. Cynthia found the subject of urination too disturbing and refused to come. Marcia was afraid that Cynthia's repugnance implied that if Sylvia were evicted and needed to live with her children, she would have to stay with Marcia. John thought perhaps his mother *should* live with Marcia, and he was angry that she was not doing her share of the caregiving. All three looked grim. If Sylvia had to develop a problem that threatened her dignity, her children felt, they had hoped the problem would have the decency to wait until she was no longer able to perceive that her dignity was under attack. Sylvia was anxious. She did not remember how often she wet herself, but she knew it was more than that one time in the bed. She did not know about the director's ultimatum, she was unaware of her fellow tenants' gossip, and she did not grasp the potential implications of her untrustworthy bladder.

But she knew in some inchoate way that she was losing control—not merely of her urine but more generally of her life—and she did not like the feeling at all.

I began with the history. When was Sylvia wet, when was she dry? Did she dribble little bits or did it all gush out? Could she tell that she had to void? If she went to the bathroom frequently, could she avoid incontinence? Sylvia was reassured by the factual questions, but she could not answer most of them. I learned that the urine poured out, it didn't drip out, and that she had never tried what we in medical-nursing jargon call a regular toileting schedule. I found out that she had no burning when she passed her water, which would have suggested a bladder infection. In addition, I learned that she had no symptoms indicative of diabetes—constant hunger or thirst—which causes increased urination and which might conceivably precipitate incontinence. Nor was she taking any new medications that might adversely affect bladder function, not even over-the-counter antihistamines. The Trumans had gotten my message about minimizing medication use when we had discussed how to avoid aggravating Sylvia's dementia. She was taking the same one-a-day blood pressure pill as when I had seen her the previous year.

Nonetheless, I was guardedly optimistic. I thought it possible, given the fairly abrupt onset of the incontinence, that Sylvia's problem was a transient one, caused by an acute, reversible condition. It was possible that she had a urinary tract infection or diabetes even though she did not have the classic symptoms of either. Her incontinence might be the only manifestation of one of these conditions. And if, after examining her for spinal cord problems or a severe form of constipation called impaction, either of which can produce incontinence, after testing her urine for bacteria and her blood for sugar, I could not find an acute cause of the incontinence, I still might be able to solve the problem. Many older women develop atrophic vaginitis, or thinning of the lining of the vagina from lack of estrogen, a process that also affects the lining of the urethra, the tube from the bladder to the outside. The thinning has the effect that urine flows when it shouldn't—and it could be significantly improved with estrogen replacement. Other older individuals, men as well as women, develop an overactive bladder. The bladder wall, which is supposed to contract only when its owner instructs it to, takes to contracting erratically. And if the involuntary contractions are strong enough and the bladder happens to be full, the urine flows out with no warning. The overactivity can be counteracted with medication, and continence may be restored.[2]

Sylvia Truman proved not to have transient incontinence. Her problem, like so many in geriatrics, was multifactorial. She had both atrophic vaginitis and hyperactivity of the bladder, neither of which, alone, was sufficient to account for her leaking, but both of which together probably were. Most likely she had had both of the underlying difficulties for some time and each had very gradually progressed to the point at which she became symptomatic.

From my perspective, the diagnoses were good news: there was treatment that had the potential to keep Sylvia dry. John was dismayed and Marcia sounded skeptical. "You mean she's going to need all this medication permanently? And one of the pills she'll have to take three times a day?"

I nodded. "If the medication works, she will probably need to stay on it indefinitely. At least the bladder pills. The estrogen she may be able to stop. And that can be taken as an internal cream rather than a pill."

Marcia cut me off. "A cream would be impossible. A pill's better." I glanced at Sylvia, who was not paying attention. She had done her best to answer my questions, she had allowed herself to be examined, and now she wanted to go home. Unless there was a nurse on site to apply the cream, it was out of the question.

"There is a potential advantage of taking the estrogen as a pill," I mused. "Some recent studies claim that estrogen might actually slow the progression of Alzheimer's disease."[3]

"The problem with the pills is the three times a day part. Mom has an attendant in the morning who helps her wash up and who can make sure she takes the morning pill. But after that, Mom's on her own. I suppose one of us could call her every evening to remind her, but I don't know how she will remember about the midday pill." We considered getting Sylvia a watch with an alarm, but the Trumans were not convinced that she would remember the significance of the buzzer. They finally agreed to try to enlist Maxine, who though only marginally less forgetful than Sylvia, really wanted to help.

In addition, Sylvia was instructed to go to the bathroom every two hours while she was awake. The motivation for this recommendation was that if she had a strong, involuntary bladder contraction when her bladder was nearly empty, little if any urine would be forced out. If her bladder was full, even a relatively small contraction would have unfortunate consequences. The idea was to keep the bladder as empty as possible, as much of the time as possible. This simple, harmless strategy would be even harder to implement since Sylvia had great difficulty learning anything new and her friends, who might remind her, were not with her all day long.

Marcia and John were discouraged, even though the treatment regimen could potentially solve Sylvia's immediate problem. They focused on the fact that it might not, and they sensed that their mother was going to need far more supervision than she currently had, if not urgently, then in the very near future. They had tried so hard to do the right thing for Sylvia, and now the image that loomed before them was of a nursing home. They looked at Sylvia, seated demurely in my office, her hands folded primly in her lap, her skirt pressed and pleated, her blouse neatly buttoned, her hair a little flamboyant (she had gone to Maxine's hairdresser). They saw her gradually transformed before their eyes: tied into a reclining chair, a shapeless housedress substituted for the suit, her hair pinned back with barrettes to keep stray strands out of her food.

Sylvia Truman's follow-up appointment was two weeks later. John brought her. He was self-employed, so his schedule was more flexible than his sister's. Cynthia was still too distraught to talk about her mother-in-law's internal plumbing. John was smiling, joking, upbeat. He had good news: he had spoken with the director of the assisted living facility, and she was satisfied that the situation was under control. Sylvia was taking the bladder medication in the morning and the evening—the midday dose had proved impossible for her to remember. She took the estrogen replacement pill once a day most of the time. Maxine and Jenny had decided that they would also benefit from frequent visits to the bathroom, so they formed the Water Closet Society. Whenever any one of them had to use the facilities, she exhorted the other members of the club to join her. Occasionally the system was disruptive, as when Maxine got up in the middle of the 7 P.M. showing of *Casablanca* and insisted that Jenny, who was seated in the front row of the lounge, take her walker and come along and that Sylvia, who had dozed off in the middle of the last row, be awakened and summoned to join the procession. And finally, as an added precaution, the aide who helped Sylvia shower and dress in the morning suggested she wear a pad in her underwear: not a full-fledged diaper, but a thick pad to catch any drops. The net effect was that the odor and the wet spots were gone.

I thought the appointment was over. Sylvia was fidgeting in her seat. I suggested that with all the talk about urinating, perhaps John had better escort his mother to the ladies' room. I would deputize him an honorary member of the WC Society. John commented that he had already fulfilled his responsibility a mere half an hour earlier. He had one more question: should they start looking at nursing homes now, and if so, how should they go about it?

Sylvia snapped out of her revery. "I don't want to live in a nursing home. I'm fine where I am."

"I don't think your son has in mind any more moves right now. And I'm glad you've decided that Silver Days Park suits you." It didn't hurt to try to remind Sylvia that she had been considerably more negative about the assisted living community when she had first moved in. "But I suspect John is thinking about the future. It's a good idea to get on a waiting list or two because a room might not become available in the facility of your choice for months or even years. If and when you do need a nursing home, you're better off going someplace that you've visited and you like, not just whatever is available."

"I'm not going to a nursing home," Sylvia repeated.

"Not now," I reiterated. "But at some point it might be necessary. Not all nursing homes are alike. They vary in terms of the physical plant and the nursing care and the activities. Many people prefer to be with other people of a similar background. They are happier if the food and the festivities are catered to their own ethnic group."

John broke in. "Mom's Italian, as you know." He turned to his mother. "I'm sure you'd like to have pasta every night. And have a priest come around every week to hear confession."

"I don't have anything to confess," Sylvia snapped. "Nobody lets me get in trouble."

John laughed. "Not even any lascivious thoughts, Mom?" Sylvia looked blank. I wondered whether she was developing trouble with comprehension, and not just with word finding. John decided to drop the subject.

"It would be a good idea to visit a few places," I told him. I handed John a list of local nursing homes, with the names and telephone numbers of their directors. I strongly suggested that he call Nancy, the geriatric social worker, to learn more about the various homes and, in particular, to discuss nursing homes with specialized dementia units. "You should go with your wife," I added. "Cynthia may have as much difficulty as your mother in getting used to the idea."

The dimples vanished from John's cheeks. He inhaled deeply and a button popped off his shirt. "Cynthia's having a hard time with all this." He gestured toward Sylvia. "She can't bring herself to talk about diapers and toilets and the rest of it. I think she'd be terrified to visit nursing homes."

"Then maybe there's something else you should do first. You and Cynthia should join a support group."

John wrinkled his nose. "I'm not the touchy-feely type. And neither is Cynthia. In fact, I'm allergic to that sort of thing."

I didn't let him off so easily. "That's what many people say. But they actually find it tremendously reassuring to meet other people who are going through something like what they're experiencing. Other families often have good suggestions, too—concrete tips about how to handle the things that are driving them crazy. Other people can report what they've tried with a parent who wanders or who embarrasses them at parties. And you'll find you have accumulated a wealth of knowledge that other family members of dementia patients might find tremendously useful. You know about day care and assisted living, and getting confused in the hospital, and now incontinence."

"I guess I'm a real expert now." John was grinning again. "I could crack jokes at the support group meetings. That might lighten the atmosphere. Apropos nursing homes, I heard a good one the other day. Bill Clinton visited a nursing home during his presidential election campaign. He walked over to an old lady in the home and said in his best Southern drawl, 'Hello, ma'am. Do you know who I am?' To which she answered, 'No I don't, but if you're having trouble remembering, I'm sure the nurse at the desk can help you.' " I burst out laughing. Sylvia was not paying attention.

I returned to my suggestion. "Seriously. You'd be a great asset to an Alzheimer support group. But you and Cynthia would get a lot out of it, too. In particular, it might be a good idea to hear about other people's experiences with nursing homes: both what it was like to move a parent to a nursing home and the inside scoop about the places around here. There's even some evidence that patients whose families go to support groups stay out of nursing homes nearly a year longer than patients whose families don't."[4]

"I'll think about it," John said as he gathered up his briefcase and jacket. "Time to go, Ma!" He woke Sylvia out of her revery and they went off for their ritual postappointment ice cream.

I did not think the Trumans would venture near a support group, and I was not convinced that Cynthia would set foot in a nursing home. I was surprised when, a few weeks later, Nancy Kingsley sat down with me in the hospital cafeteria and told me that John, Cynthia, and Marcia had all come to see her.

"They had been to an Alzheimer support group meeting and were ready to start exploring nursing homes. Apparently they met a woman who had been a full-time time caregiver for her demented mother. The woman had been on the verge of collapse from stress and fatigue, and was ecstatic now that her mother was safely ensconced in a special care unit. She had felt overwhelming guilt at the prospect of institutionalizing her mother—evidently she had promised her father on his deathbed that she'd never 'put Mom away.' But she had come to the realization that she actually was not taking very good care of her mother—at least that's what she felt—she simply did not have the patience or the professional distance or the resources to provide what they could give her in the nursing home."

"Did you find out the name of this terrific place?" I inquired, a bit skeptically.

"As a matter of fact, the Trumans were so excited that they had already rushed off to visit. It's called Golden Acres, and it's brand-new. They still have empty beds, so the Trumans thought they'd better act quickly. They have a great patient-to-staff ratio and an architect designed the building to be bright and cheery with circular corridors for the patients who pace, and elegant but water-resistant furniture for those who piddle. They have an activities director with experience in dealing with Alzheimer's disease and a psychiatrist on staff who visits biweekly to monitor and adjust medication. It sounds pretty good, but it's part of a proprietary chain with a mediocre reputation. I'm not sure whether the Trumans were impressed because it's clean and shiny—and half empty—or whether it's really a decent place."

"Not smelling of urine is a plus," I reminded Nancy. "And it sounds as though they have incorporated most of the promising ideas used in other dementia units."

The concept of a special nursing home (or a wing in a larger nursing home) exclusively devoted to the care of the dementia patient is fairly new. Unfortunately, little rigorous testing has been performed to determine whether outcomes are better in special care units than in conventional nursing home settings. The ideal study, in which incoming nursing home residents are randomly assigned to either a regular floor or a dementia floor, is very difficult to conduct. And defining and measuring the impact of care is also problematic: should investigators study whether residents take fewer psychotropic medications and wear fewer physical restraints, whether they scream less, or whether their families are more satisfied than their counterparts on the regular floors? The existing studies are largely descriptive—they simply state what was done differently and assert that it made a difference.[5]

Another related approach used by some of the few large nursing homes, those with more than two hundred beds, is to group residents according to their physical and mental condition. In this model, those with dementia live together on one floor, and those with physical problems necessitating extensive nursing care but with no intellectual problems— including people with strokes or multiple sclerosis or Parkinson's disease—live together on another floor. In some very large institutions, further refinement is possible: among patients with dementia, those with aggressive, disruptive behavior are segregated from those who sit quietly all day. Attempts are made to staff each of these very different floors with personnel experienced or interested in the kinds of problems on that unit.

Designating part or all of a nursing home as a special care unit is clearly a good marketing strategy. In the increasingly competitive environment of nursing homes, those facilities that call themselves "special" have an edge. But all nursing homes care for a clientele that is disproportionately demented—in surveys of the nursing home population, upwards of fifty percent have dementia—regardless of whether they advertise expertise in the field.[6] And all nursing homes are under pressure to improve the care of their demented residents. Thanks to 1990 federal government regulations, nursing homes are required to minimize their use of physical restraints. They are compelled to document carefully the need for antipsychotic medication and to demonstrate ongoing surveillance for evidence of side effects in those residents in whom such drugs are used. The rules arose from journalistic accounts of abuses in nursing homes, which in turn led to a series of recommendations by the prestigious Institute of Medicine.[7] These included such basic common-sense recommendations as allowing families to visit at any time and requiring a standard nurses' aide training program as a prerequisite for certification.

Other regulations governing nursing homes affect the care of all residents, but are particularly important in protecting the rights of individuals who are unable to speak for themselves. A state-appointed ombudsman must have access to all nursing homes to gather information periodically and hear complaints, improving nursing home accountability. Minimum standards for staff:patient ratios help ensure that residents receive adequate care. In large measure due to the implementation of these recommendations, the quality of care in nursing homes has improved considerably.

My beeper went off, terminating our lunch. I made a bet with Nancy about Sylvia Truman—I said I didn't think her family would institutionalize her quite yet. Sylvia was not ready, and I did not think Cynthia was ready. Nancy disagreed. She said that John, for all his bravado, was very anxious about assisted living. He didn't think half an hour a day of personal care was sufficient for his mother. He thought the director was inexperienced. He felt as though the only people consistently looking after Sylvia were her newfound friends, who were only slightly better put together than she was. Nancy disclosed that Marcia had called her up to tell her she was getting divorced and starting a new job—and that if she had any more stress in her life right now she would fall apart.

I was stunned. The Trumans were the best-adjusted, most supportive family of an Alzheimer's patient I had encountered. If the burden of the responsibility for Sylvia's well-being was too much for them to take, how could anyone be expected to deal with it month after month, year after year?

The social worker won the bet. Two weeks later, Sylvia Truman was back in my office for a preadmission physical examination—a medical check-up was part of the application process for nursing homes. Her regular physician was out of town, and they needed the form taken care of immediately. Golden Acres had had twenty empty beds when they visited; now it was down to six. Four of the six were reserved for women. They had visited three other places and had rapidly developed a sense of what to look for.

"One of the homes smelled," John began. "In another one, most of the residents were in bed. This wasn't ten at night—it was ten in the morning. I asked if it was naptime, but the nursing director told me no, it was just the patients' usual routine. I figured some of them liked sleeping late, and some might have asked to go back to bed, but they couldn't *all* have an excuse for remaining in bed. Especially when the other places we went to had everyone up and dressed by eight A.M. and sent them off to activities by nine. And a third one looked kind of cozy: it was a big old mansion, with nice wallpaper and even a few paintings on the walls—not the usual institutional flavor—but the staff turnover was phenomenal. They'd had three nursing directors in a year, and the average tenure for the nurses' aides was four months. There was obviously something very wrong with the management at that one. By comparison, Golden Acres was paradise."[8]

"Which doesn't mean it was perfect," Cynthia interrupted. So she had gone along on these visits. "We're not that naive. The big question is whether it will still seem like a good place when it's been around for a year, when it's full, when the furnishings begin to fade and need repair or replacement. We're just hoping that the philosophy they've adopted will prevail and will make all the difference. Most of the nursing homes we visited were clearly staff centered: everything was organized to make life easier for the nurses and the nurses' aides. The design was intended to simplify the lives of those who worked there, with a central nursing station and long corridors, like a hospital. Bathing times and eating times—even bedtimes—were set up for the convenience of the nursing home personnel. One home we saw was built to cater to visitors: everything looked nice, at least on the ground floor. There was a lounge with a grand piano, a garden at the entryway, a gift shop so families could buy something at the last minute if they had forgotten to bring along a present. There was even a little restaurant for visitors. But the residents didn't ever use any of those facilities. It was all for show, things to appeal to outsiders. The residents sat tied into their chairs, lined up along the halls, upstairs and out of view of the casual outsider. Golden Acres is patient centered. They try to figure out how the residents want to lead their lives, which isn't always easy, and determine staff schedules and activities accordingly. Of course they have certain constraints, too—"

"Like money," John cut her short.

"And we don't know whether they really have enough nursing assistants or whether their in-house training program is any good. But at least they're committed to trying."

I had never heard such a long speech from Cynthia Truman. The business of dealing with her mother-in-law had not been easy for her. Even with her husband's exuberance and involvement, a large share of the burden managed to find its way to the women in the family.[9] Once Cynthia had come around to believing that Sylvia needed to enter a nursing home, she had done her homework to find the best available option and there was no turning back now.

"When is all this going to happen?" I asked, wondering if Sylvia had any idea what was afoot.

"As soon as you mail in the results of the physical and we provide a bit more information about Mom's financial situation. Probably in another couple of weeks. She'll be private pay at first, though after a year she's going to run out of money. She'll have to go on Medicaid—the nursing home will help us file the application—and then Medicaid will pay for the nursing home."[10]

"I'm not going into a nursing home." We all turned to Sylvia, who had not shown any signs of paying attention to the conversation.

"It's just for a visit." Cynthia practically pounced on her mother-in-law. She was not going to brook any opposition at this point. "It's time for a change of pace—like a vacation, time to go someplace different."

"I don't want to." Sylvia looked as though she was going to cry. I didn't know whether she understood that her move was not planned as a mere visit, or whether she was overwhelmed by the recognition that her life was being run for her. She sounded like a child. John, who had done his best not to infantilize this sad, broken person who was, after all, his mother, put his arm around her.

"It's okay, Mom. Just give it a try."

There was a moment of silence while they all pulled themselves together. Sylvia decided not to resist; Cynthia struggled to overcome any doubts she had about deceiving the old woman; John stayed very still, allowing his mother to feel his devotion and his affection.

John disrupted the tableau. "One more thing. Mom will need a doctor to go out to see her at Golden Acres. Her regular doctor does not make nursing home visits. They gave us a couple of names of doctors who have patients at Golden Acres. But we were wondering if you'd be willing to take Mom on."

I looked at the three of them—scared, guilty, and imploring by turn. I looked up at John. "I guess this is your chance to get rid of us," he said, smiling. It was a shrewd comment. With Sylvia, I acknowledged, I had only the weakest of ties. I didn't think she remembered me from visit to visit. I didn't think it mattered much to her who her doctor was. Obviously it did make a difference, even if Sylvia could not understand such things, that some physicians were more attuned to geriatric issues than others, and some physicians were more comfortable at discussing limitation of treatment near the end of life than others. But clearly, John and Cynthia, and to a lesser extent Marcia, had become my patients over the preceding two years, and I felt a responsibility toward them. "It's not that," I began. Suddenly I could not proceed with a litany of excuses, explanations. "Sure, I'd be honored to take care of Sylvia at Golden Acres."

So it was settled. Two weeks later, I received the call that Sylvia was a resident at the Golden Acres Nursing Home and that I had forty-eight hours to get over there to see her. No matter that I had just performed a physical examination in my office, the results of which they had in hand, as it had been a prerequisite to her admission; the regulations called for a doctor to "admit" the patient, on site, within two days of her arrival. I chose to skip grand rounds at the hospital, the weekly lecture attended by a large fraction of the medical staff, which this week was on new radiologic techniques. I risked interrupting Sylvia's breakfast, but I would only minimally disrupt my day.

Golden Acres presented a cheery face to the external world. It was nicely landscaped, with large automatic glass doors to allow wheelchairs and walkers easy access. The lobby was attractive as well, featuring a lounge in which residents and their families could congregate, overlooking a small but sunny courtyard. The information desk was tucked off inconspicuously to the side, conveying the impression of an apartment building rather than an institution. Sylvia Truman, I learned, was on corridor C on the second floor.

Corridor C was circular, as Cynthia had mentioned, permitting residents to pace endlessly without getting lost and without confronting the frustrations engendered by a dead end. There were a few nice touches: an indoor "porch," replete with an awning and rocking chairs, to simulate an outdoor terrace; special washable carpets in the halls instead of slippery tile. It was brightly lit and the signs on the rooms were large and easy to read, designed to help residents orient themselves by labeling rooms with placards saying "bathroom," "nursing station," and "dining room." But in other respects, the floor looked like the other nursing homes where I saw patients. The residents were of course all old—the mean age must have been eighty-five. Several were lined up in the hall, securely belted into their wheelchairs, dozing or watching the world go by. One lady constantly called out, "Susan!"

"I'm not Susan," I told her as I walked by, hoping the human contact, however brief, would be reassuring. She switched gears. "Ellen, Ellen," she cried.

Sylvia was still in the dining room. She had a bib tied around her neck. Jam was smeared around the corners of her mouth. A few crumbs had managed to find their way into her hair. I said hello to her, but she stared blankly at me. "I'm Dr. Gillick," I reminded her. "I saw you in my office a few times." Still no recognition. "John brought you. John and Cynthia," I elaborated, hoping to gain credibility by referring to her family.

Her eyes brightened momentarily. Then she glared at me angrily. "Did you tell them to put me in here?"

"No," I answered, though perhaps it would have been better had she blamed me for her situation, rather than her children. "But I did say I would check on you here." She resumed her breakfast, and I decided to familiarize myself with the system at this nursing home—meet the head nurse, look at the medical record, find the order book.

I chatted briefly with the nurse, explaining my business, commenting on how spiffy the nursing unit appeared. "It does look nice," the matronly Irishwoman agreed. "But I'm afraid the residents don't much care how it looks, though their families do. The residents care about how the aides treat them, and it's no better than average in that regard. I was promised that we would have time for special in-service education for the staff on caring for people with Alzheimer's." She put the emphasis on the second syllable. "It's a bit difficult when half the workers don't speak English." She was describing what was a reality in most nursing homes: the aides were at the bottom of the totem pole; they did the most difficult work for the lowest pay. They were poorly educated and often non-English speaking.[11]

An aide approached the desk as we spoke. "She's in her bed," she reported without making eye contact. The nurse was relieved that our conversation had been interrupted. Perhaps she sensed that she had divulged too much. "Come with me," she commanded curtly. "I'll show you to Mrs. Truman's room. It's a very nice room, overlooking the garden."

Sylvia had been escorted to her room and was sitting motionless in the one chair. She had a bed, a night table, and a closet. There were a few built-in bookshelves, on which were perched pictures of John, Marcia, and assorted grandchildren. A faded black-and-white photo of Sylvia and her husband on their wedding day formed the centerpiece of the display. The wallpaper was pale blue with tiny white flowers. A colorful hand-crocheted blanket lay neatly folded at the foot of her bed. A calendar hung on the wall, the date circled. A clock radio and an unopened letter were the only ornaments on the night table. Apart from the pictures, the room could have been in a motel—except that in the middle of the room was a curtain, partitioning off the half belonging to Sylvia's roommate.

"How are you doing?" I asked jovially, but feeling slightly apprehensive.

"Fine," she answered mechanically.

I walked over to her and went through the motions of a brief examination: I took her pulse and listened to her heart and lungs. The yield from checking the heart and lungs of an asymptomatic individual like Sylvia was extremely small. Moreover, I had gone through a standard exam a mere two weeks earlier. I decided that what I really should do—which the nursing home had not requested on its form—was a minimental status exam.

"I'd like to see how your memory is," I said. "These are just routine questions, all right?" She nodded. I repeated the brief, standard exam I had given her at the time of the initial geriatric consultation, testing memory, language, visuo-spatial skills, and abstraction. Her score was 14 out of a possible total of 30, down from 20 three years ago.

I was saddened to have demonstrated so starkly how much she had declined. But her abysmal performance was in its way reassuring: it justified the move to the nursing home. Not that a score on the mental status exam correlated perfectly with functioning in daily life. And indeed with consistency, structure, and a lot of reminders from her friends Maxine and Jenny, plus telephone calls from her children, Sylvia had managed remarkably well in her apartment at the assisted living community. Watching her struggle to remember, to find words, seeing her fail as she tried to draw a plain clock, I realized what Sylvia's children had recognized for some time—her intellectual abilities were fading fast.

As I mumbled some platitude about how inconsequential my memory questions were, Sylvia's roommate stormed into the room.

"Get out of my chair, you hag!" she screamed. Sylvia cringed.

"This is Sylvia's chair," I stated matter-of-factly. "Let's find your chair." I pulled back the curtain separating the two halves of the room, but Sylvia had already gotten up meekly and moved over to her bed. Her roommate, however, had lost interest in the chair and had started rummaging through Sylvia's drawers.

"Why don't you come with me?" I gestured to Sylvia, and escorted her into the hall. I then proceeded to the nurses' station to request help for Sylvia's neighbor. As I wrote the obligatory note in the medical record and orders for Sylvia's care, much as I would in the hospital, her roommate charged down the hall, invective pouring from her mouth.

Two other residents were using the circular hallway like a racetrack, doing laps. Another woman was seated in a "geri-chair," a padded seat with an attached tray that served as a restraint. She had removed her shoe and was pounding rhythmically on the tray. Her nurse cleverly substituted a bedroom slipper for her oxford to turn down the volume of the banging. A distinguished-looking man dressed in a suit came over to the nurses' station and politely asked for directions to the travel agent. The nurse pointed in an arbitrary direction, the man thanked her, and he started off on his fruitless quest. Like a rat on a treadmill, I thought, as he disappeared from view. One woman who had been sitting quietly in the corridor, apparently watching the comings and goings of the other residents with interest, suddenly began taking off her clothes. A nurse's aide tried to help her put her blouse back on, but she was pushed away. The aide shrugged her shoulders and left. A minute later the aide tried again, with no greater success. A second nursing assistant brought a blanket

from the resident's room and draped it over her, a valiant
effort that was effective for a few seconds until the resident
cast off the blanket.[12]

When I left the nursing home, the man in the suit had just
completed one circuit. Evidently he had forgotten about the
travel agent. He shook his head disapprovingly as he passed
the bare-chested woman, and muttered that the police ought
to arrest the ladies of the night. The head nurse had given up
trying to distract Sylvia's roommate and was on the phone
with the woman's physician, attempting to get an order for
tranquilizing medication. Sylvia was still sitting quietly in the
hall where I had left her, fear and incomprehension in her
eyes. She had exchanged an environment in which she
was among the least capable for one in which she was among
the most intact. I wondered whether the move had been a
mistake.

Back in my office, I called John Truman to discuss his
views, as her health care proxy, about the kinds of medical
interventions that would be appropriate for her, should she
develop a new medical problem.

"You've seen her?" he asked. I indicated that I had just
come from the nursing home. "The roommate situation is
intolerable." I had to agree. Not all individuals with dementia
also exhibited aggressive behaviors, and for a woman like
Sylvia to share quarters with someone who was hostile and
perhaps violent was as much a mismatch as the pairing of a
quietly demented woman with a cognitively intact roommate.
The goal of an institution such as Golden Acres was that
behavior viewed as bizarre among the healthy but commonplace among the demented—pacing, disrobing, perseverating—
.would be readily tolerated. If residents were allowed to walk
the halls, bang their shoes, and ask the same questions
repeatedly without censure, they would be happier and the
community more peaceful than if they were forcefully
restrained. The problem was that certain kinds of behavior
had a traumatic effect on others. For the sake of communal harmony, something had to be done about Sylvia's
roommate.

John was surprisingly optimistic. "They're going to move
that other woman to a private room. Hopefully Mom's new

roommate will be more like her—confused but quiet. So how did you think she was doing?"

I assured him that his mother was much as she had been a few weeks earlier, though I thought she was bewildered by some of the antics on her floor. I mentioned that I was startled by just how much her thinking had deteriorated.

"She really does fit in, you know," John said. Many families had tremendous difficulty accepting the diagnosis of dementia in their relatives. They persisted in denying that anything was amiss, even after it had become blatantly obvious to the rest of the world. They blamed Dad's forgetfulness on normal aging. They excused his repetitiveness on the grounds of hearing loss, claiming he had not heard their answers to his question the first six times he'd asked. They argued that his socially inappropriate behavior was just a longstanding personality trait. The Trumans, once the word *dementia* was out in the open, had not resisted the truth. If anything, they were relieved to learn that Sylvia's peculiarities were neither her fault nor theirs, that they were caused by her disease. They were also, I suspected, pleased that her diagnosis was strictly medical rather than psychiatric, since mental illness carried a stigma for them. Better an illness of the brain than of the mind—at least until such time as psychiatric disorders could more unequivocally be identified as neurologic disturbances.

I returned to the reason for my phone call. "Now that I'm your mother's primary care doctor, I need to get some sense from you, as her health care proxy, about how to proceed should Sylvia become ill."

John knew immediately what I was getting at. "We don't want her on any machines. Mom would never have wanted that."

"So if her heart stopped beating, you would not want attempts made to start it up again—"

He interrupted me. "If her heart just stopped—if she died in her sleep—it would be the best way for her to go."

"CPR—cardiopulmonary resuscitation—is only rarely successful for someone like your mother, particularly in the nursing home, where they don't have all the apparatus available in a hospital, or personnel trained to use that stuff." I felt John needed to hear that his decision made sense on technical grounds as well as on ethical grounds; quality of life was not the only relevant consideration here; also significant was the fact that CPR in the nursing home was as close to being futile as any medical intervention ever was. Virtually nobody from a nursing home with multiple chronic illnesses, including dementia, survived a cardiac arrest. In those rare cases in which survival had been reported, the individuals typically suffered brain damage from lack of oxygen or were in other ways left significantly more debilitated than previously.[13]

Perhaps I was reassuring myself; John was very comfortable with my designating his mother's status "do-not-resuscitate," or DNR. "Even if it worked half the time, we wouldn't want it. She's eighty-five and her mind's going. She'll be lucky if she has a massive heart attack."

I moved on. "You said you wouldn't want her on machines. I assume you mean a ventilator to breathe for her if she were in a coma and were unable to breathe on her own." He grunted assent. "But suppose she had a major pneumonia and a respirator could tide her over until antibiotics and her own immune system kicked in. What would you think about using high-tech interventions on a temporary basis?"

This was a possibility John evidently had not considered. "All I know is that I wouldn't want her hooked up to all kinds of things indefinitely."

"But how about for a few days, or a week, or whatever we agreed upon at the time, with the understanding that if the machine for breathing, for example, didn't work—if Sylvia did not improve in the expected period—it would be discontinued."

"Can you really do that?" John was incredulous. "I've read about too many cases where the doctors or the hospital insisted on going to court if the family wants to disconnect a machine. Not that I have any objection to people going to court—that's what keeps a lot of my colleagues in business. I know all too well that it's a long-drawn-out business, and it can be very unpleasant, too. Not to mention the fact that much of the time these legal battles are decided after the patient's dead." He laughed. I enjoyed John's willingness to make fun of his own profession.

* * *

Both the courts and medical ethicists agree that competent patients—patients in possession of their mental faculties—have a clearly established right to refuse treatment. The right to decide what is done to a person's body is grounded both in the common-law right of self-determination (the basis for the informed consent doctrine) and in the constitutional right of privacy.[14] Over the years, court cases have revolved around numerous types of treatment refusal—including blood transfusions, dialysis, and feeding tubes. In each instance, judges have ruled and ethicists have concurred that individuals are free to decline any and all proposed interventions, regardless of their likely benefit, and on whatever grounds they choose, provided they are capable of understanding the consequences of their decision.[15]

If competent patients cannot be compelled to undergo medical treatment that they do not want, then surely incompetent patients, those whose ability to think and reason is sufficiently impaired that they cannot themselves make meaningful choices, should not be required to submit to all possibly effective therapy, regardless of the pain and suffering entailed. And so the litany of cases involving competent patients' right to refuse treatment has been repeated for incompetent patients. Again and again, judges have ruled and ethicists have argued that surrogate decision makers, acting on behalf of incompetent patients, can refuse precisely the same interventions that the patients could have refused, had they been able to speak for themselves. The courts have repeatedly affirmed the legitimacy of surrogates' refusal of chemotherapy, dialysis, and cardiopulmonary resuscitation.[16] And finally, in the first "right to die" case brought before the U.S. Supreme Court, the justices upheld the acceptability of withdrawing artificial nutrition and hydration for an incompetent patient, asserting that being fed through a tube was conceptually identical to undergoing any other medical procedure, and that surrogates may authorize the withholding of any and all medical interventions.[17] The one twist to the Supreme Court ruling was its determination that state legislatures may impose standards to which surrogates must adhere: that is, they may, if they choose, require that surrogates supply evidence that their wards would in fact not have wanted the particular treatment. Alternatively, state legislatures can decide that appointing a proxy automatically confers the right—and the responsibility—to limit treatment. Some legislatures have passed family surrogate laws, which appoint a surrogate if the patient has not already done so, based on a specified prioritization of the next of kin. In many states, even without family consent laws or a legally designated proxy, the patient's immediate family is assumed to have the right to make medical decisions for an incapacitated relative.

Implicit in this discussion is the moral and legal equivalence between withholding and withdrawing treatment. Although John Truman was right that physicians and families often feel that these two acts are psychologically distinguishable—physically unhooking a ventilator or removing a feeding tube feels different from failing to hook up the ventilator or insert the feeding tube in the first place—careful scrutiny suggests there is no meaningful distinction between acts of omission and acts of commission. If a patient has stated clearly and unequivocally that he would not wish attempts at resuscitation should his heart stop, and his heart does stop and he dies, is that situation morally any different from a patient who has made the same request but who has a cardiac arrest in a hospital where the doctors and nurses are unaware of his request and therefore start CPR—but discontinue their efforts when the patient's wife comes crashing into the emergency room, frantically waving her husband's extremely explicit advance directive? Arguably, withdrawing treatment that has been unsuccessful in achieving its goals should be less objectionable than never even trying in the first place. That is, the concern that removing treatment is "killing" a patient but failing to initiate treatment is "allowing to die," does not make sense. In both cases, the assessment is made that the patient has what will probably be a lethal condition, and that the burden of the treatment to the patient is too great to warrant its use—whether initial use or continued use. Or, in those cases where the patient is comatose and cannot be said to find anything burdensome because he cannot experience pain or suffering, the treatment is withheld or withdrawn because it has not been, and is unlikely to become, successful in producing its intended goal: restoration of the individual's personhood.

* * *

The upshot of my conversation with John Truman was that he agreed to a DNR status for his mother, but not to any other limitations of treatment. He decided it would be reasonable to have her on a respirator, in an intensive care unit, in order to treat a pneumonia or a heart attack, if those few days of treatment served to allow her to return to her current condition. He did not believe that the discomfort of this kind of aggressive treatment was so great as to preclude its use. And he was not prepared to assert that the quality of his mother's life was so poor that she would be better off dead. I wondered what it would take for him to change his mind.

CHAPTER 8

Alzheimer's Disease in the Eyes of America

Whenever I saw Sylvia Truman in the office or the hospital or the nursing home, I saw her through the lens of medicine. I tended to focus on her deficits: I was forever characterizing, naming, and measuring what she could *not* do: she had trouble with words, she had difficulty finding her way, her short-term memory was shot. The nurse and the social worker who form part of the geriatrics team at my hospital, in advising her family, were more likely to capitalize on the capacities she still had—Sylvia could read and comprehend simple directions, so labels on her drawers that said "Underwear" or "Sweaters" enabled her to find her clothing; Sylvia's dexterity was good, so if she had her pills laid out in a special dispenser, with each day's supply clearly marked, she was unlikely to overdose on her medications. My job in large measure was to ascertain what skills she had lost and whether her functioning in a given domain had declined since the last time I saw her.

Because Sylvia looked physically like the woman he had known all his life, John saw her as the same person she had always been, with a few loose screws. By contrast, because I had never known Sylvia Truman when she was cognitively intact, I did not see a whole person with a few missing pieces; I principally saw the holes. When John looked at his mother, he perceived the continuity with her earlier self. But both of us, despite our different starting points, saw Sylvia filtered through another, common lens. Our emotional reactions to her, the fears and anxieties she engendered, derived to a considerable extent from the way our society sees dementia.

The desire to explain life's misfortunes is deep-seated in the human psyche: diseases with no known cause and no effective treatment make people decidedly uncomfortable. If science cannot provide an explanation, the popular imagination will. These commonsense theories reflect deep-seated beliefs about what makes people get sick; they often reveal as much about prevailing conceptions of good and evil, of upright and dissipated living as they do about pathophysiology. They frequently embody widespread fears that have little to do with the disease in question but are merely projected onto it. Tuberculosis, for example, one of the leading causes of death among young adults in the nineteenth century, was extensively mythologized by poets, novelists, and to some extent the general public. In the struggle to make sense of a senseless disease—a disease that struck people who were in their prime, people who were sufficiently virtuous that to regard their illness as punishment was absurd—tuberculosis came to be seen as an expression of the inner self. The illness was attributed to the sick person's personality, in this instance to the positive features of his or her character. The victims were to blame—but for being too emotional. TB was thought to arise from too much passion, afflicting those who were excessively sensual and overly sensitive. Moreover, contracting TB, rather than undermining those qualities, was believed to intensify them. TB sufferers became *more* seductive and *more* creative. In the imagery of the late nineteenth century, the "tubercular look"—a pale, emaciated appearance—was considered attractive.

A society that was striving to come to terms with the Industrial Revolution's new ideal man, the ruthless entrepreneur, quite naturally viewed the passionate and sensitive person as a misfit. At the same time, the ambitious capitalist was a not altogether appealing person, whereas the sensual, emotional individual was. But the dreamer, the poet, was set up for failure in society. What better way to explain his failure than by linking his personality to the development of the almost uniformly fatal illness tuberculosis? No matter that not all TB sufferers were sensitive and spiritual, and no matter that not all delicate, artistic people developed TB. Conjoining a mysterious illness and a particular personality type served a useful purpose for the nineteenth-century mind.[1]

Cancer, similarly, is sometimes attributed to personality in contemporary American society. Despite the considerable media attention devoted to carcinogens in the environment, to the role of cigarette smoking and high-fat diets in causing cancer, despite all the attention to oncogenes (genes associated with particular cancers), the perception prevails that some people are "cancer prone" by virtue of their character. In contrast to the once prevalent model of TB, cancer is thought to develop in people who are sexually repressed and inhibited, who are unspontaneous, and above all, who fail to express emotion. If TB was formerly thought to stem from too much passion, cancer is now thought by some to come from too little. Perhaps this construct represents a backlash against the same successful, domineering bourgeois who was once thought to be immune to TB because of his personality. This societal ideal, while economically successful, perhaps turned out to be personally unsuccessful. The distaste for the bureaucrat, the technocrat, and the political insider is symbolically linked to a major twentieth-century disease with unknown etiology—cancer. In an attempt to make psychological sense of an often lethal disease involving unchecked cellular growth and of a society that rewards productivity over creativity and compliance over innovation, the two become metaphorically merged.[2]

Any common disease "whose causality is murky, and for whom treatment is ineffective, tends to be awash in significance."[3] Understanding the significance attached to a disease may tell us a great deal about the society that develops the metaphors. At the same time, the metaphors shape the reality experienced by the sufferers from the illness: it matters tremendously to an individual with TB, cancer, AIDS, or Alzheimer's disease, not just what his physical symptoms are, but also how he is perceived—and therefore treated—by his society.

What does Alzheimer's disease look like to most Americans? How does it fit in with prevailing notions about aging, disease, and disability? Alzheimer's is described in popular writing as "the silent epidemic" and "a funeral that never ends." It is referred to as "the disease of the century" and as a "dread disease." The effect of the disease on families of the afflicted is captured in the title of the most widely read self-help manual about Alzheimer's, *The 36-Hour Day*.[4] It is a disease that "robs families of their loved one," that "steals the mind," and that is a "creeping, lurking, wily, and thieving travail that infiltrates elderly lives uncontrolled and uncontrollably."[5] The devastation wrought by Alzheimer's is also described in economic terms—it is the "third most expensive disease," by some calculations, after heart disease and cancer. Alzheimer's effects are quantified by using mortality statistics—some describe it as the fourth most common cause of death—and by citing the numbers of nursing home beds filled by dementia patients (probably close to 1 million).

Moving beyond these sound bites to a fuller understanding of the meaning of this "dread disease" is not easy. Many would argue that America is far too diverse and multicultural to hold a single popular view of dementia. Nonetheless, I think we can draw some conclusions about the *dominant* view. Pockets of Americans may hold deviant views, but we can delineate a majority view from a survey of articles in the news media, of television programs, and of magazines and books targeted to the elderly themselves.

Old People in the News

The graying of the population is a fairly common subject for newspapers. Journalists are particularly intrigued by the rising number of centenarians. Only three thousand Americans were over one hundred years old in 1960; in 1995 the number reached fifty-four thousand, and the projection for 2050 is that there will be 2.7 million.[6] Aging is not just an American phenomenon or a Western phenomenon: the age structure of the entire world is changing. Over half of all the elderly, or 200 million people, live in the developing world, where they comprise 4.6 percent of the population. The most recent life expectancy figures, like census data, grab the media's attention. In 1995, an eighty-year-old American woman could expect, on average, to live another eight years.[7] The reason for the intense interest in the numbers, of course, is not just how remarkable they are, but also their economic implications. More old people translates into unprecedented numbers of retired people, all drawing on Social Security. As a result, Social Security has overtaken defense as the largest item in the federal budget.[8] This means that retirement at age sixty-five is becoming increasingly untenable, both economically and psychologically. An individual who retires at sixty-five can expect to spend a quarter of his life retired.[9] The demographics are also newsworthy because they spell trouble for the Medicare program. Medicare Part A, which covers hospital care, home care, and skilled nursing care, is paid for by the Hospital Insurance Trust Fund, which is expected to become insolvent by 2002. Medicare Part B covers physician services, outpatient hospital services, and laboratory fees. The majority of its funding comes from the U.S. Treasury, so it has a profound, direct effect on the federal budget. Spending on Medicare Part B is growing 50 percent faster than expenditures on Part A. Overall, spending on Medicare is growing at 10.5 percent per year.[10] Given all these gloom and doom forecasts, it is not surprising that reporters are eager to find a fix. Hence, dominating the news stories about old people are four claims: 1) aging in general and physical disability in particular are largely preventable through good nutrition and exercise; 2) mental exercise can eliminate or at least diminish much cognitive disability; 3) the individual with Alzheimer's loses his humanity so the real victim is the caregiver, but fortunately, 4) a cure for Alzheimer's is just around the corner.[11]

The idea that a special diet and physical activity might delay aging is not new. The sixteenth-century Venetian Luigi Cornaro attributed his longevity—he ultimately lived to age ninety-eight—to abstinence, temperance, and regimentation.[12] American health reformers of the nineteenth century regarded nutrition and exercise as the keys to all medical ills, including the disabilities associated with old age. The current resurgence of interest in diet and fitness reflects prevailing notions of individual responsibility: we have a strong desire to believe that each person can shape his own destiny. A good, vigorous old age, in this view, does not require enormous government expenditures or elaborate genetic engineering. All it requires is that every person take his destiny into his own hands—those who live right will live well.

For the first time in history, there is scientific data that exercise and diet *can* make a difference in health and well-being. Aerobic exercise decreases the risk of heart disease, which is one of the major causes of illness and death in old age. More generally, it leads to lower mortality and slows down the development of disability.[13] The elderly can also improve their muscle strength, even in their nineties, using an individually tailored program of weight lifting, and these gains are directly translated into better functioning in daily life.[14] In the realm of diet, adequate calcium intake promotes strong bones, which in turn decreases the risk of osteoporosis, which in turn lessens the chance of fractures. Older people must take in enough calories and protein to maintain their strength. On the other hand, they must avoid overeating, since obesity contributes to the development of conditions such as heart disease and diabetes.[15]

Asserting that exercise and diet have a modest role to play in producing a vigorous old age is a far cry from proclaiming they are the elixir of youth. Unfortunately, much of the reporting on old age in the media exaggerates the benefits of regular exercise and a wholesome diet. Vitamin B_{12}, for instance, is clearly essential for a variety of physiologic processes: the bone marrow requires B_{12} to make red blood cells, the nervous system needs the vitamin for both thinking and walking. But to maintain, as one journalist did, that B_{12} deficiency leads to "senility" and "paralysis" is misleading.[16] Insufficient B_{12} is one of the causes of reversible dementia, and patients with dementia should certainly have their B_{12} level checked with a blood test. But *most* people with dementia do not have B_{12} deficiency as the cause, and most people who are low in B_{12} do not have dementia. Even those people who do have both dementia and inadequate levels of B_{12} turn out only rarely to improve their cognition with replacement of B_{12}—not because the replenishing is undertaken too late, but because they prove to have *both* B_{12} deficiency and Alzheimer's disease. The assertion that eight out of ten chronic illnesses are "influenced by nutrition" should not be taken to imply that 80 percent of the degenerative diseases associated with old age are preventable through proper diet.

Other dietary supplements, such as vitamins C and E, are touted as reducing heart disease and mental decline, respectively, despite the absence of solid evidence for either claim.

One feature story, for example, describes a researcher at St. Louis University who is in his eighties. "At 87, Dr. Max Horwitt," the article begins, "is old the way people dream of being old. Horwitt's body is strong enough for a daily paddle around the swimming pool. His mind is sharp enough to continue his research on aging at St. Louis University." Dr. Horwitt is reportedly unsure of the reason for his success, but he takes antioxidants and he follows a low-fat diet.[17]

Always eager to report on any connection between exercise and successful aging, the news media picked up on a study published in the *New England Journal of Medicine* about predicting disability. The study itself involved examining over a thousand people seventy-one and older, and then following them for four years. Of those still alive in four years, the ones who initially had the lowest scores on physical performance tests had four to five times the risk of subsequently developing disability. The journalist concluded that if physicians can identify which older people are at greatest risk of disability, they will be able to "give treatments that prevent or postpone the onset of those impairments."[18] Unfortunately, prediction does not imply prevention. Moreover, poor performance might well be associated with underlying disease that is already insidiously impairing function—rather than merely with a lack of physical fitness.

Not only is exercise widely believed to prevent disability, it is also held up as the secret to *longevity.* When Jeanne Calment of France turned 120 years of age, dozens of journalists and scientists flocked to her nursing home in the hope that they would discover the clue to her survival. The key to longevity has eluded innumerable fortune seekers, from Ponce de Leon, who sought the Fountain of Youth, to the formidable though eccentric Russian scientist Elie Metchnikoff, who injected himself with ground animal testicles in the belief that this concoction would prolong his life. Jeanne Calment, who lived to be 122, herself recommended "a smile as a recipe for long life,"[19] but the professional judgment was that the key to a long life is limiting alcohol, forgoing smoking (though Calment herself quit smoking at age 117), and above all, exercising regularly.[20]

The twin leitmotifs of prevention and individual responsibility as the keys to avoiding physical disability in old age were dominant themes at the 1995 White House Conference on Aging, which was widely covered in the media. Delegates agreed that elderly Americans "must take charge of their health earlier to avoid the decline and infirmity that are often part of the aging process." A report issued by the conference, entitled "Putting Aging on Hold," argued strongly that diet, exercise, and other preventive measures could solve the health problems of old age. Not only was prevention touted as essential to improving the well-being of the elderly, it was also alleged to be the key to maintaining the solvency of the Medicare trust fund. Regular exercise and sound nutrition, by some calculations, could lead to a savings of $260 billion in Medicare expenditures over a five-year period.[21]

Individual behavior *can* make a difference, but the image in the popular press of old people jogging their way to health and casting off their canes and walkers is excessively naive and simplistic. The same holds true for mental disability in old age.

Intellectual Calisthenics

If nutrition and exercise can stave off physical deterioration, mental gymnastics, in the popular view, can prevent cognitive decline. Assisted living facilities, such as the apartment complex where Sylvia Truman lived for a time, are lauded in the media not only because they allow privacy and independence, but also because they maintain "self-reliance." The "operative rule" of aging, according to newspaper accounts, is "use it or lose it."[22] There *is* evidence that institutions such as nursing homes can produce "learned helplessness"—people who are prevented from exercising any control over their lives, even in domains they have the capacity to influence, become more dependent than other, comparable nursing home residents who are allowed to make choices in their daily lives.[23] But this intriguing observation about the potent effects of institutionalization is far more complex and subtle than simply "use it or lose it."

The belief that mind work can prevent mind disease crops up in reports of the "nun study." Members of several convents agreed to periodic mental status testing in life and autopsies at death. Preliminary results from this ongoing study were recently published. A characteristic popular account of the study begins with the reassurance that dementia is not an inevitable concomitant of aging. "Only" 37 percent of the ninety-four autopsies performed to date revealed evidence of Alzheimer's disease. Since not all the nuns in the group being followed over time have died yet, this figure may well turn out to be close to the 48 percent found in the largest, most carefully conducted investigation of the prevalence of dementia in those over eighty-five. Since even a 37 percent rate might be worrisome, the reporter offers more reassurance: "Currently scientists have a rule-of-thumb theory about Alzheimer's that may or may not be borne out in the nun study: the more mentally active you are, the less likely Alzheimer's is to strike you."[24] Ironically, the next scientific paper to come out of the nun study alleged that those nuns who wrote very simply when they were in their twenties were destined to develop florid Alzheimer's a half century later.[25] Other work has shown that education is inversely associated with the risk of Alzheimer's disease. Whether this statistical relationship stems from the fact that the better educated are more likely to exercise their minds, or whether it arises from different occupational exposures in those with varying levels of education, or whether it simply reflects better test-taking ability in people with extensive schooling is unknown.[26] What is clear is that the belief that thinking prevents Alzheimer's is wishful thinking.

Another twist on the claim that individual behavior can positively affect cognitive capacity is the claim that "intellectual ability is maintained . . . as long as [the elderly] stay active in their private lives."[27] While early studies of cognitive function in old age seemed to suggest such an association, subsequent larger studies have shown that the relationship is more complicated. Dementia is correlated with *physical* illness (strokes and heart disease, for instance) and those who are sick tend to lead less active lives.[28] Ironically, the one arena in which individuals can have an enormous impact in staving off dementia—the treatment of high blood pressure—is largely ignored in the popular press. There is now substantial evidence that high blood pressure is the culprit in a large proportion of dementia other than pure Alzheimer's: in multi-infarct, or vascular dementia. This variety, which causes about

40 percent of all dementia, and perhaps more since some people have a combination of several types, may be preventable through tight control of blood pressure. If doctors diagnose high blood pressure and prescribe sufficient medication, and if individuals take their pills even when they feel perfectly well, vascular dementia can probably be largely eliminated.[29]

Not to Worry: A Cure for Alzheimer's Is Imminent

Even though we are led to believe that disability in general and Alzheimer's in particular are largely preventable, we are also encouraged to think that if we nonetheless develop Alzheimer's, a cure is imminent. Major breakthroughs in medical research are another favorite topic for newspaper articles dealing with the elderly. Unfortunately, many of the dramatic new advances turn out not to be as promising as they initially seemed.

Increasingly, families who bring in their forgetful older relative for a geriatric assessment, much as Sylvia Truman's family brought her to see me, demand an apolipoprotein E test, which they have read allows prediction of who will develop dementia. The discovery of the *APOE* connection (see Chapter 2) was immediately picked up by the press. This simple and relatively inexpensive blood test (at the going rate of $100 to $200 the test is not cheap but far less expensive than the $500 to $1,000 cost of an MRI) was alleged to allow prediction of which older patients were destined to develop full-blown Alzheimer's. The test could "help doctors decide which patients should be treated aggressively to slow or halt progression of the devastating disease."[30] Unfortunately, of those who test positive, only 61 percent later develop Alzheimer's (as do 24 percent of those who test negative). Put differently, if individuals with a positive test are led to believe they have or will get Alzheimer's, 39 percent will be misinformed. Likewise, a quarter of people with negative tests will be falsely reassured that they do not have and will not get Alzheimer's. Moreover, while physicians would like to aggressively treat people with mild symptoms to slow the disease, they currently have no approved drug to prescribe for this purpose.

In addition to learning that a *predictive* test has ostensibly been developed for Alzheimer's, the public has been told that a *diagnostic* test is available: people with a memory disorder can ostensibly be told whether they have Alzheimer's or not, even when they have only mild symptoms. The "test" is actually a combination of two tests: blood *APOE* typing and positron emission tomography (PET scanning), a sophisticated form of brain imaging that reveals the function and not merely the structure of the brain. While this pair of tests is promising, it has by no means been shown to be reliable.[31] And, as with tests alleged to show who will eventually develop Alzheimer's, early knowledge of one's fate mainly serves to produce a prolonged period of anxiety.

Predictive tests and early diagnosis are encouraging developments—or might be if they were accurate—but even more exciting would be a real cure. Headlines such as "Brain Graft Help for Alzheimer's Shows Promise" suggest that implantation of brain tissue is likely to be a viable therapy for Alzheimer's disease. However, the relevant research cited is a study in rats. Scientists deliberately damaged that part of the rat brain involved in making the neurotransmitter acetylcholine, the biochemical that is deficient in people with Alzheimer's disease. Scientists then implanted cells that could produce acetylcholine into the brains of those rats and found that rat function improved, in activities such as running mazes. This is fascinating stuff—but its applicability to people with Alzheimer's disease in the near future is highly questionable.[32]

Most people probably realize that there is neither a cure nor effective treatment for Alzheimer's, but they are repeatedly told that "Alzheimer's disease is beginning to surrender its terrible secrets." The discovery of the gene on chromosome 14 that causes 70 percent of early-onset, inherited cases of Alzheimer's led to the comment that "armies of gene researchers around the world are closing in on some of the causes of the disease."[33] It is certainly the *hope* that the discovery of the gene will lead to unraveling the cause of the destruction of cells in Alzheimer's disease, and will result in the ability to slow or halt that destruction. At present, however, little more is known about this gene than that it codes for a protein that forms part of the membrane, or outer layer, of brain cells. Both the normal function of the protein, and the role played by the abnormal variant (manufactured from a mutant gene) are mysteries.[34]

The belief that a cure for Alzheimer's is imminent is no mere figment of the journalistic imagination: some scientists in the field are tremendously upbeat about the immediate clinical implications of their work. Allen Roses, Professor of Neurology at Duke University and a discoverer of the importance of *APOE*, has predicted that "within ten years we will have a pill that prevents Alzheimer's disease."[35] Other researchers foresee that a means of *slowing the progression* of Alzheimer's disease *might* be developed in the next five to ten years. Researchers on the cutting edge of the Alzheimer's field are in general ebullient about the strides that have been made over the past few years, as well they should be—the pace of research has been extraordinary. But the *scientific* goal of understanding is often distinct from the *clinical* goal of effectively treating real people with real problems.

Alzheimer's Is Grotesque

The final message from the media about aging is that Alzheimer's is a devastating, dreadful disease. The people for whom it is most disastrous are portrayed as the caregivers, the estimated 25 million people "juggling the demands of their job and families while trying to meet the often overwhelming needs of elderly mothers, fathers, husbands and wives." If the numbers currently involved in taking care of elderly families are enormous, they are only going to get larger. It is the oldest old (those over eighty years old) who are the most likely to have major physical and mental problems—50 percent require significant assistance to survive day to day. Right now there are 3 million Americans over eighty; by 2030 the number is expected to be 9 million, and by 2050 it is expected to reach 19 million. As "70 million baby boomers come face to face with the demographic reality, somebody is going to have to take care of their parents, and that somebody is most likely going to be them." The job, far from being a natural filial responsibility, is uniformly depicted as burdensome: "It's just the start of another day in the frustrating, solitary, often depressing struggles to take care of the woman who once took care of her" starts a four-part magazine series on caregiving.[36]

The plight of the adult caregiver who must deal with Alzheimer's in her mother or father is depicted as particularly heart-wrenching. She has to change her mother's diapers or give her father a shower. She has to provide assistance to someone whose life she regards as not worth living.[37] Our society values self-sufficiency, so we have little tolerance for the dependent and accord little respect to those who take care of them. Only rarely are the media descriptions of a demented older individual and his family balanced: written both from the perspective of the old person and of the caregiver, portraying both positive and negative features of reality. One moving account of a ninety-year-old woman with Alzheimer's living in a retirement home comments that the woman, Mildred, looks for her mother every day. Her son, who visits her daily, "has given up explaining reality. What's real is what's in her mind, he says. Some days he is her son, some days her brother. [He] knows he can never unbend her mind, so he straightens her twisted stocking instead." For the most part, Mildred is not unhappy and her son is usually cheerful. "Some things survive," the author reports. "For Mildred it is the beauty instinct." But on some days, it is too much for her upbeat son to bear, and he is quoted as telling his wife, "If I end up like that, take me out and shoot me."[38]

Alzheimer's disease can be so horrible that some caregivers resort to murder, as in the "typical" murder-suicide scenario in which a man caring for his demented wife kills her and then turns the gun on himself.[39] Suicide and physician-assisted suicide are also prominently featured "solutions" to the horror of Alzheimer's disease. Dr. Jack Kevorkian's first client was Janet Adkins, a woman alleged to have mild Alzheimer's. Her case received widespread media attention, though suicide is rare among individuals with true Alzheimer's.

Victims of Alzheimer's disease do not just sit quietly in their rocking chairs, journalists remind us. They may be uncontrollably violent: a child visiting a nursing home was actually attacked.[40] Clearly this kind of behavior does occur: Alzheimer's disease *can* be unrelievedly grim. But absent from description in the popular press is the caregiver who finds her role fulfilling, who has had a longstanding close relationship with her mother and delights in helping her at the end of her life. The reality is that children of demented parents often care in a way that no hired aide possibly can, precisely because they remember their parents as they once were. Children or spouses are often the best caregivers, not out of obligation or necessity, not merely because there is no one else to do the job or no money with which to pay someone else to do it, but because they are motivated by *love*.[41] The popular conception of Alzheimer's disease does not include the old person who is cheerfully oblivious to his dementia. If any attention at all is paid to the perspective of the demented person himself, it is to his deficits rather than his residual strengths. The prevailing view is that the individuals whose intellectual calisthenics were insufficient to stave off Alzheimer's disease can expect a horrible existence, as Alzheimer's "spreads tendrils of damaging neural fibers and islands of protein, called plaque, through the human brain, suffocating memory and destroying personality as it slowly kills."[42]

What Is a Good Old Age and How Does Dementia Fit In?

The image of aging on television, in retirement magazines, and in books about growing old is not substantively different from the picture presented in the news media: aging is nothing to be feared since all the decline and disability stereotypically associated with getting older are preventable. For those people who do not take matters into their own hands to avert disease and disability, medical science is certain to come to the rescue in the near future.

The predominant picture of old age in the entertainment industry is of gray-haired, wrinkled versions of young adults. By and large, only the robust elderly make it to prime time (and not very many of them) because most television programming assumes there is nothing moving or amusing or inspiring about living with disabilities, whether physical or cognitive. As one poll of television writers, directors, and producers concluded, TV is a form of escapism for viewers; they have no desire to think about unpleasant nuisances such as death or disability.[43] Hence those television dramas that include older people typically feature tough, vibrant elders who embody the venerable tradition of rugged individualism.

While the media capture the issues associated with aging, magazines and books targeted to the retired population discuss what they take to be a good old age. The key theme here is that old age is—or should be—a time to pursue individual fulfillment. Gone are responsibilities to family and job; what remains are the time and the opportunity to cultivate the self. Popular literature commonly suggests consumption as the means of self-actualization, in the form of travel, entertainment, clothes, and cars. Hence *Modern Maturity*, the periodical of the American Association of Retired Persons, and its British counterpart, *Retirement Choice*, feature movie reviews and articles about traveling. The advertisements, which create a very graphic portrayal of the good life, chiefly push retirement communities, luxury cars, and exotic travel. Even the magazine *New Choices for Retirement Living*, which acknowledges that not all elderly persons are vigorous and which does address topics such as terminal illness, dementia, and death, paints a vivid picture of the good life in its advertisements: large, powerful cars confirm the elders' vitality, including upscale models from Buick, Mercury, and Cadillac. There are a few mundane travel specials, such as discount rates offered by several United States motel chains, but no spot is too remote to consider. A single issue of the magazine advertised a trip to Hawaii, a "celebrity cruise," a world cruise, and special travel sections from the Malaysian Tourism Promotion Board and the Tourism Authority of Thailand. All told, out of thirty-nine half-page or larger ads, fifteen (37 percent) were for travel. When old people are not on the road or the open sea, they are encouraged to spend their time in an upscale retirement community such as a "golf villa" in Florida.

To have the energy to travel—or to stay home and swim or play tennis in the country club atmosphere of a retirement village, the older set must exercise and eat well—the same message as in newspaper accounts of new truths about aging. Hence both feature articles and advertisements promote exercise (a fleece jogging suit, a NordicTrack WalkFit machine, and a video on strength training all made their appearance in one issue of *Modern Maturity*), and nutrition (from cranberry juice to a chromium supplement). The prevailing image of the body in most retirement magazines is that it is a "machine which can be serviced and repaired. . . . The array of products and techniques advertised cultivate the hope that the period of active life can be extended and controlled into a future where ultimately even death can be mastered."[44]

The proliferating books on how to stay young or how to make the most of the retirement years take as their starting point the claim that old age is a period of "continued growth."[45] Betty Friedan, in her best selling book *Fountain of Age*, exhorts older people to find new outlets for their creativity: they should write books, take up painting, develop new skills, even embark on new careers. They should also cultivate new relationships since intimacy is a critical ingredient of successful aging—whether in the form of romantic love or close friendship.[46]

While the popular books on aging focus on individual fulfillment, they also acknowledge that *meaning* often derives from community involvement, from giving as well as growing. Friedan comments that most of the "vital" older people she has known applied their "wisdom" to the "problems of our society." She recognizes that "we need to evolve new ways of working and learning—no longer defined by career—to give purpose to our days and to keep us part of the human enterprise." Ken Dychtwald, founder of the Senior Actualization and Growth Exploration Project (SAGE), echoes her sentiments. He discusses the need for older people to "give back" to the surrounding society, drawing on their experience and knowledge. The elderly, he suggests, can and do provide meaningful assistance to the young as advisers, to their peers as health care advocates and tour guides, and to their more disabled counterparts as shopping assistants or companions.[47]

The trouble with this exhilarating view of aging is that it leaves out dementia and disability entirely. The authors of these inspirational works, perhaps because their focus is primarily on the "young old," people in their sixties and seventies, barely acknowledge that there is such an entity as Alzheimer's disease. Dychtwald maintains flat out that "there is no such disease as senility." He claims that study after study "has shown people who stay active and intellectually challenged not only maintain their mental alertness but also live longer." Gail Sheehy, in her book *New Passages: Mapping Your Life Across Time*, adds her voice to the chorus of enthusiasts for the "discipline of daily mental exercise." She offers a new twist, that psychological attitude is the key to determining "the quality of duration of our third age." Belief that we will remain free of dementia, in short, is a self-fulfilling prophecy.[48] Friedan chooses to minimize the significance of Alzheimer's by stressing the fact that only 5 percent of Americans over sixty-five have dementia—quietly omitting the observation that nearly 50 percent of those over eighty-five are afflicted. She would like to believe that "only in the last months of life do most people suffer disabling deterioration," neglecting to recognize that the duration of Alzheimer's disease is typically seven to ten years. And finally, she mistakenly thinks that most of those diagnosed as having dementia actually are cognitively intact. The 60 percent of those in nursing homes who are "supposedly suffering from irreversible senile dementia, Alzheimer's disease," she believes, have mental deterioration caused by institutionalization, which "can be mistaken for senility."

The growth and fulfillment model of aging represents the positive pole of what historian Thomas Cole calls the "dualism" of aging. The critics of ageism, debunking the myth that all old people are unproductive, sick, and "senile," have created a new stereotype of the old person who is "healthy, sexually active, engaged, productive, and self-reliant."[49] The true challenge is to find meaning in old age *despite* physical and cognitive decline, and to accept the inevitability of death.[50] While the demented person can enjoy life—he may well derive pleasure from listening to music or eating a good meal—he cannot "grow" in the sense of doing new things. Learning a new hobby is precisely what the individual with dementia *cannot* do. She might still be able to form relationships, as Sylvia Truman did with her roommate in the nursing home. She may be able to make a contribution to society, whether by reading stories to preschoolers, or by fleshing out the description of World War I in her grandson's history book through her personal oral history. But the rosy image of aging in books and magazines, like that in the news media, leaves little solace for old people with dementia or, for that matter, with other chronic illnesses.

The Origins of the Contemporary View of Aging

The overwhelmingly positive image of aging, with its minimization of the role of dementia, is in large measure a reaction against earlier, uniformly gloomy depictions of old age. At the turn of the century, when Alzheimer made his critical discoveries, aging was synonymous with deterioration and decay. Precisely because the human organism was *expected* to wear down over the years, causing loss of function in all domains, including cognition, Alzheimer's disease was presumed to be distinct from the mild cognitive decline often found in old age. From the Civil War through the first decade of the twentieth century, this negative image prevailed. Victorian morality, whether in Europe or transplanted to the American continent, regarded independence, health, and success as the cardinal virtues. Control over one's body was seen as the means of pursuing wealth, ambition, and happiness. "The decaying body in old age, a constant reminder of the limits of self-control, came to signify precisely what bourgeois culture hoped to avoid: dependence, disease, failure, and sin."[51] Since it was patently obvious that dependence and disease did exist, commonly, in old age, the Victorians chose to explain away those people who appeared to challenge their theories by simply blaming them for their failure to age well. They were presumed to be "shiftless, faithless, and promiscuous" and therefore "doomed to premature death or a miserable old age."[52]

In the United States between 1909 and 1935, social reformers and academic gerontologists gradually transformed the Victorian view. Old people, they argued, were *all* sick, weak, and debilitated, through no fault of their own. Because they could not be expected to be independent—and because their inadequacies were deemed to be a natural consequence of aging—social programs were essential to support them. Professional expertise and scientific knowledge, in the form of people such as social workers, physicians, and physical therapists and institutions such as nursing homes and hospitals, were promoted as the solution to the problem of aging.

Since the 1960s, the pendulum has swung back to the Victorian view, complete with the caveat that the flowering anticipated in the retirement years is contingent on the elderly taking charge of their lives. Old people must eat right, exercise, and stay intellectually and socially active. These claims about what can and should be achieved in old age are consistent with prevailing beliefs about what is important in life, at any age.

Dementia in Our Day

For most Americans, the meaning of life is entirely self-defined: the specific goals of a good life are a matter of personal preference. Being free, in fact, means "being left alone by others, not having other people's values, ideas, or styles of life forced upon one, being free of arbitrary authority in work, family, and political life."[53] Not only do Americans uphold the right to choose their own values and standards, but they also expect each individual to have the opportunity to get ahead, to become his own person. Getting ahead, usually measured in terms of material success, is what life is taken to be about. Typically, this fulfilment of one's potential is achieved primarily through work. It is principally through your job, paid employment, that you can expect to "make something" of yourself. This leaves homemakers and retired people in the lower echelons of society; it leaves demented people in the subbasement.

Americans may have lost much of their faith in the ability of government and economic growth to solve social problems, but not in the ability of the individual to make something of himself. If anything, the declining respect for American institutions has redoubled the belief in the primacy of the individual. American culture today is "a society in which the individual can only rarely and with difficulty understand himself and his activities as interrelated in morally meaningful ways with those of other, different Americans. Instead of directing cultural and individual energies toward relating the self and its larger context, the culture . . . urges a strenuous effort to make of our particular segment of life a small world of its own."[54] With this sort of radical individualism, meaning does not stem from a person's position in the community—as, for example, in societies such as India in which the elderly are valued for their experience. All that matters is the exercise of individual choice. Not only is the autonomous individual expected to derive meaning apart from family or community, he or she is also expected to find a purpose in life outside of any national or religious tradition.

Given that the ideal of American life remains the self-reliant, self-creating individual, it is no wonder that the portrait of old age in the news media, on television, and in retirement magazines conforms to this standard. The contention that exercise and diet can prevent physical decline implies that even a very old person, by continued application of good habits, can maintain his independence. The assumption that dementia can similarly be avoided by using one's mind, by remaining socially active, is likewise a critical component of the contemporary worldview. In a society in which a technical fix is thought to be available for most problems, surely a medical fix will soon exist for dementia (in those relatively rare instances when Alzheimer's disease cannot be willed away).

The widespread belief that Alzheimer's disease is dehumanizing follows logically from the central role of self-reliance in the American psyche. The loss of the ability to shape one's life is the quintessential feature of Alzheimer's disease. This disorder, which progressively impairs memory, judgment, reasoning, and the ability to learn new things, which makes it difficult to figure out how to get dressed and impossible to solve everyday problems, strikes at the heart of the American ideal of control. John Wayne and Horatio Alger are still folk heroes: John Wayne because his single-handed toughness and integrity allowed him to subdue the forces of evil around him, and Horatio Alger, because his perseverance and hard work enabled him to become a millionaire. Alzheimer's disease is exactly the sort of condition that Americans find hardest to deal with—a common disorder over which we have absolutely no control.

For the person with Alzheimer's disease, the domain over which she can exercise choice is tremendously restricted.

Even when Sylvia Truman retained the cognitive capacity to figure out that she would like to shop for a new pair of shoes or eat out in a restaurant or go to a movie, she had lost her ability to carry out her plan on her own. She was dependent on others to realize her wishes. Even when her cognition deteriorated to such an extent that her family had to make decisions for her about her medical care or moving to a nursing home, she was still able to make some choices— about what she ate, or what she wore, or whether to take a nap.[55] While the limited sphere in which she could exercise choice meant a great deal to her, the consequence of her eviscerated autonomy was that she was viewed by society at large as a half-person.

Because American culture regards the capacity for control as essential to personhood, journalistic accounts of Alzheimer's disease exude pity and dread. The writers' sympathies lie with the caregivers, the "hidden victims" of the disease: the people whose day lasts thirty-six hours and who describe Alzheimer's as a "funeral that never ends." This attitude fails to take into account the fact that many individuals with Alzheimer's disease, from its earliest to its most advanced stages, are unaware that there is anything wrong with them and can derive a great deal of satisfaction from their lives. Sylvia Truman, when she first moved to the assisted living facility, appreciated the convenience of having meals served three times a day, acknowledged the efficiency of living in a small apartment instead of a large house, and grudgingly admitted the desirability of on-site social activities. But she vehemently denied that she could not live in her own home. She continued to have strong likes and dislikes, both in companions and in dinner entrees, and to experience the full gamut of human emotions, from joy to despair. Even the nursing home residents with advanced dementia with whom Sylvia was housed when she entered Golden Acres Nursing Home appeared to enjoy eating, music, and, above all, the compassionate contact with another human being. Only in the very last stage of Alzheimer's disease, in which people can no longer swallow food and respond fleetingly, if at all, to others, are all vestiges of personhood gone, leaving only a physical shell.

Sylvia Truman was frustrated at her inability to remember and to do things for herself once she progressed beyond the early phase of believing she had no limitations. But her disappointment at her growing dependency abated as she adapted to her new state, much as someone with a stroke can adapt to using a cane, and someone with macular degeneration can adjust to diminished vision. The reconciliation process is especially difficult with dementia, precisely because of the societal premium placed upon self-reliance. Sylvia nonetheless came to accept her deficits—not in a conscious, explicit way, but gradually, over time. Our challenge as a culture is to find a way to reciprocally accept and respect those with dementia, despite their inherent dependency.

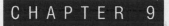

CHAPTER 9

Midnight

Thursdays were my days for nursing home visits. On the first Thursday of the month I made it a habit to go to Golden Acres, where I had built up a small panel of patients—usually three or four at any given time.

On this particular trip, I decided to save Sylvia for last. I had begun to find seeing her depressing. She never recognized me. She was no longer able to make conversation—she could simply answer yes or no to questions, and I could not depend on the veracity of her answers. She no longer appeared frightened, but neither did she ever look happy.

The first patients I visited were Mildred and Milton Schwartz. They were among the few patients at Golden Acres who had entered as a couple and who shared a room. They both had dementia—hers was probably Alzheimer's disease and his was most likely due to multiple small strokes. She was otherwise perfectly healthy. In addition to his strokes, he had had several heart attacks and developed cramps in his legs when he walked, because of poor circulation. If it were not for the dementia, Mildred would have been a robust elder, able to engage in vigorous physical activity, with no limits on what she could do. Milton, in contrast, had severe, diffuse atherosclerosis of the blood vessels nourishing his brain, his heart, his legs, and probably many other bodily parts as well. On some days he suffered from angina, chest pain due to lack of oxygen to his heart; on other days it was the claudication (pains in his legs) that limited him. But despite his problems, the couple were inseparable. Mildred was outgoing, sociable, always smiling. Milton followed her around, dutifully attending meetings of the garden club and the ceramics workshop. Mildred could not remember anything that had been taught previously about potting plants or glazing bowls, so the instructors in each activity were perpetually starting from scratch. This meant that for Mildred each class was a revelation, an inspiration, though the source of the awe and wonder she experienced was the same from class to class. Milton did not share his wife's joy, but he seemed satisfied that he was fulfilling his matrimonial obligation, despite his failing memory, of which he was vaguely aware.

The couple were very protective of each other, which I found endearing. This morning Mildred told me that Milton had been complaining of abdominal pain. He denied it—or couldn't remember—and I had no idea whether the pain had occurred that day or the previous day or perhaps weeks earlier. The nurse on the Schwartzes' nursing unit found a note in Milton's medical record indicating that he had been out of sorts the previous evening. He had vomited once after dinner, gone to bed early, and been fine since. I examined his abdomen, inquired about his bowels, and concluded that whatever it was, it had vanished as mysteriously as it had arrived, and I assured the pair that I doubted it was serious.

Mildred had no complaints, nor was her nurse worried about her. I listened to her heart and lungs in a perfunctory way, as a symbol of my concern for her physical well-being, and watched her bound off her bed when I had finished. She became frustrated trying to find her handbag, I observed, but Milton noticed it perched on his night table. "I wonder what it could be doing there," Mildred mused, as though she had never confused her night table and his, but chuckled loudly at what she took to be one of life's many puzzles. I wished the Schwartzes well and headed to the nursing station to enter a brief note in each chart. For Mildred: "No new medical problems. On exam, looks well. Lungs clear. Heart without murmurs. Able to dress and get out of bed without assistance. Participates in nursing home activities. Cheerfully unaware of her deficits." And for Milton: "Only new problem since last visit is one episode of abdominal pain. Vomited after dinner last night. No nausea, no diarrhea, no further pain. No constipation. On examination looks frail but comfortable. Abdomen soft, obese, with normal bowel sounds. Self-limited problem of unclear etiology. Otherwise stable." I moved on to visit Annette Simonson.

I found Annette seated in a wheelchair in front of her bureau, all the drawers open, tossing articles of clothing onto her bed. A pile of scarves and underwear lay on the bed; a few knickknacks were scattered on the floor. "I can't find it!" Annette wailed.

"What are you looking for?"

"I'm looking for, I'm looking for . . ." Her voice trailed off. I was not sure whether she couldn't remember the word or whether she had already forgotten what she had lost.

"Let's pick up a few of these things before you trip on them," I suggested.

"No, no, I have to, I have to . . ." Tears filled her eyes.

"Would you like the nurse to help you?"

"Aren't you the nurse?"

"No, I'm Dr. Gillick. I just came by to check on you."

"Isn't that nice!" She beamed.

"Does anything hurt you?" I asked, seizing the opportunity to divert her from her hopeless quest.

"No, yes, I think so."

"What bothers you?"

"Everything!" She began to cry again. I looked at her hands, misshapen from rheumatoid arthritis, and wondered whether her pain was entirely emotional, or whether the arthritis still bothered her. I took her hands in mine, one at a time, and palpated each deformed joint. Annette was smiling again. I concluded that her anguish was not caused by her rheumatologic problems.

They had, however, spelled the beginning of the end of her. She had been a devoted first grade teacher in a parochial school for forty years. She had never married: her life had been the school, her students. When she wasn't preparing her lessons or correcting papers, she was directing the class play or creating magnificent costumes for the children. Her hobby was writing children's stories, which she illustrated herself. She never succeeded in publishing any of these but gave her most polished products to her students as prizes for outstanding work.

In her early sixties, Miss Annette, as her pupils called her, had been forced to retire. Her hands had become so weakened from arthritis that she could barely hold a piece of chalk. She had missed more and more days of school because of incapacitating flares of her disease, which caused swelling of her knees and pain in her wrists. She had tried all the available therapies, from high-dose aspirin to gold shots, but finally had to give up teaching. Generations of fond students visited her at home, bringing home-baked breads and pastries, and, more important, news of their accomplishments to cheer her. But she had lost her raison d'être, and though the rheumatoid arthritis ultimately burned itself out, leaving her joints deformed but pain free, her mind never recovered.

It was in the setting of this chronic, low-level depression that her dementia had insidiously begun. Annette ceased being able to name every student who had ever sat in her class, she forgot the telephone numbers of her closest friends, and she could no longer compose children's stories, even using a tape recorder. She cried at the slightest provocation, tears reflecting the vast sadness she felt at all she had lost.

When I started seeing Annette Simonson at the nursing home, she no longer remembered what she had lost. She did not know she had been a teacher; she did not recognize any of the books she had created. But her overwhelming grief persisted. She was like a child who cried because she was separated from her mother in a crowd—except that Annette did not know who was missing and would never experience the relief of reunion.

As Annette could not report any symptoms, I consulted with her nurse. No, the nurse assured me, Miss Annette had not had any new problems in the month since I had last seen her. She slept poorly at night, which, the nurse observed thoughtfully, seemed to exacerbate her daytime confusion. Would I reconsider a sleeping pill? I had tried sedatives before, but Annette had become excessively lethargic, even with the lowest possible dose of a medication that was rapidly metabolized and excreted. I nodded at the nurse appreciatively—she seemed genuinely distressed that Annette's baseline misery intensified at night, and was not merely interested in quieting her for the benefit of the night staff. I promised to order trazodone, a sedating antidepressant that might help

Annette sleep and would simultaneously provide another opportunity to tackle her weepiness pharmacologically.

Annette Simonson's sense of hopelessness rubbed off on me: I left her feeling powerless in the face of dementing illness. Yet seeing her was less depressing than seeing Sylvia Truman, because I had never known Annette when she was a whole person. What I knew of her past I knew from the social service notes in her chart and from a brief conversation with her nephew, her only surviving relative. I could imagine the woman she had once been: firm, demanding, tough on the outside but mellow within. Sylvia, on the other hand, I could remember from an earlier time. She was already diminished when I first met her, but her pride, her sense of humor, her resolution, had still been evident. The woman I had come to visit had been distorted almost beyond recognition by the disease that was destroying her mind.

Sylvia was sitting in the hall when I arrived on C corridor. She had become one of the ladies who spent most of the day in a chair, alternately watching and dozing. Her day was punctuated by meals and an afternoon nap. She sat in on bingo but could no longer play unassisted. She sometimes watched the evening movie on the nursing home's large-screen television, but she seldom could follow the plot and usually fell asleep before it was over. She had to be washed and dressed: left to herself, she neglected all but her face, put her clothes on backward, and left the buttons undone. Sylvia could still feed herself if her food was cut up for her and she was reminded what to do with her fork and spoon.

"Hello, Sylvia," I said.

"Hello," she responded dutifully. "How are you?" She had not lost her social graces.

I reached over to take her pulse. She shoved me away. This was a new development, I thought. Previously she had pushed me away only when she was delirious, after her hip fracture. "Leave me alone," she barked.

I tried to distract her. I attempted my old trick of mentioning her children. "John?" she echoed, after I mentioned her son's name. "I went to the, with the, and John," she announced. I couldn't make sense of what she said.

"How about Marcia? Has Marcia been to see you?"

"Yes. She came." I wondered whether this was accurate. "She came with my mother." I concluded it wasn't.

"Okay, Sylvia." I put my arm around her. "Have a good day."

I wrote my note about Sylvia in her medical record. "Continues to decline mentally. Memory and language especially affected. No acute events or motor weakness to suggest a recent stroke. Will recheck thyroid functions and vitamin B_{12}. Condition most consistent with moderately severe Alzheimer's dementia."

It was time, I thought, to speak with Sylvia's health care proxy about further limitations of care. In the four years I had known her, she had been remarkably healthy, apart from the dementia. Her only hospitalization had been for her hip fracture; her only other acute illnesses, several upper respiratory infections. At eighty-six, odds were she would develop some disease in the near future. The leading causes of death in her age group were heart disease, stroke, cancer, and pneumonia. Not everyone with those illnesses succumbed to them; but did John want his mother to live on if she had a heart attack or came down with pneumonia?

Most advance planning is restricted to discussions of limiting treatment in the setting of imminent death. Living wills, for example, are usually of the form: "If my death is imminent, I would not wish . . ."[1] Not only does advance planning—whether by patients when competent or their surrogates when they are not—usually focus on treatment in the most dire circumstances, but it also customarily addresses only the most invasive treatments. The one kind of limitation of treatment that doctors routinely ask about is whether to attempt resuscitation in the event that the heart stops. That is, physicians ask whether they should try to revive a person who has died—a practice that can be dramatically successful in a person who has an irregular heartbeat after a heart attack, but that is almost never successful in the very elderly with multiple chronic conditions. In the nursing home setting, as I had discussed with John Truman when Sylvia first entered Golden Acres, the probability of successful resuscitation is perilously close to zero.

Apart from cardiopulmonary resuscitation (CPR)—chest compressions to mechanically keep the blood flowing through

the heart while electric shocks and intravenous medications
are administered, plus artificial respiration either via mouth-
to-mouth breathing or through a tube put down the trachea
and into the lungs—there are many other interventions used
in sick, older people that can legitimately be withheld if they
are felt to be too burdensome. Some of these, such as dialysis
for kidney failure and chemotherapy for cancer, are included
in detailed intervention-specific advance directives.[2] But even
when physicians broach the advisability of employing invasive
technology, they often take for granted that these treatments
would be withheld only in patients who, if not terminally ill,
are irreversibly comatose. In fact, both unambiguously invasive therapy, such as mechanical ventilators, and procedures
that are arguably less uncomfortable or hazardous, such as
intravenous fluids and antibiotics, may be viewed as excessively burdensome in an old, chronically ill individual. Commonplace medical interventions such as nasogastric tubes or
pacemakers are frequently riskier in debilitated older people
and they are also less likely to be effective than in their
younger counterparts.[3] Likewise, they are riskier in people
with dementia, since brain failure poses just as much a threat
to the integrity of the entire person as does heart failure or
kidney failure. Individuals with advanced dementia are unable to understand what is happening to them. They cannot
cooperate with their nurses and physicians, whether by lying
still, taking a deep breath, alerting an attendant that their
intravenous has become dislodged, or simply leaving tubes in
place. Both diagnostic studies (X rays, endoscopy, electro-
cardiograms) and treatment modalities (surgery, medications, exercises) work best when conducted in a participating
rather than in a passive or protesting patient. Sylvia Truman
was in a phase of her dementia in which she could no longer
be a partner in her medical care but instead would be the
reluctant recipient of any tests or treatments that I might
prescribe. It was these other intermediary forms of treatment
that I wanted to discuss with John Truman.

I never initiated a conversation with Sylvia's son about
which limitations of care other than CPR might now be
appropriate for Sylvia; John brought it up himself. I found
a message from him one afternoon, after rounding on my
hospitalized patients. "Call John Truman," the pink slip

instructed me. "Important but not urgent." I wondered what was amiss. I had received no calls from the nursing home, so Sylvia's nurse apparently did not believe she was ill. I ticked off a few possibilities in my mind. John was moving his mother to another nursing home; he had heard of a new miracle treatment for Alzheimer's disease; he was worried that her medications were adversely affecting her.

My speculations were all wrong: John was quite satisfied with his mother's nursing home (he had minor grievances but no reason to believe another facility would be any better); no cures for Alzheimer's disease, real or imagined, were being touted in the media; and Sylvia was taking only one medication, her antihypertensive. John proved to be quite upset, but what was distressing him was Sylvia's roommate.

The bed next to Sylvia's had been home to a succession of occupants. The belligerent woman who had been Sylvia's first roommate had been moved into a private room, as promised. Her second roommate, a wizened woman no more than four feet six, had seemed perfectly content at Golden Acres, but her daughter had found the home wanting and moved her to another nursing home after a few weeks. Rumor had it that the other home had not proved satisfactory either and that the daughter had ultimately taken her mother home with her. Sylvia's third roommate seemed to be a good match: she was quiet, like Sylvia, demented to roughly the same extent, and even shared Sylvia's Italian heritage. For Sylvia, sharing a room had been traumatic—she had not been compelled to cohabit with anyone since she had moved out of her parents' home at age eighteen, bequeathing her bedroom to her sister. For the next sixty years, she had cheerfully slept in the same room as her husband, but she had chosen him, and he her. Moreover, they had had ample space for privacy: even their first apartment boasted a kitchen and a living room. While the assisted living community in which Sylvia had had an apartment consisted merely of a bedroom, sitting room, and bathroom, at least those had been her own. Now suddenly only her bed was uniquely hers. But if she was destined at this late stage in her life to have an arranged marriage—to another woman, no less—Angelina Nicolazzo was an ideal match.

Angelina had moved to the United States from Italy when

she was nearly seventy. Her husband had died, and she was the youngest of six siblings, with ten years between herself and the next oldest. Her brothers and sisters were either dead (three of them) or ailing themselves and unable to serve as companions or caregivers. Her four sons all lived in America—two in New York, one in Boston, and one in Chicago. They got together on the occasion of Luigi's twenty-fifth wedding anniversary. Salvatore, the eldest, decided that their mother should join them in the States. Giancarlo, who was by far the wealthiest, said he could not agree more, but he could only help financially since he did not have a wife into whose care his mother could be entrusted. He had had a wife, two in fact, and was planning to marry an aspiring actress half his age in another month, but the job of looking after Angelina should fall to a mature woman, well versed in the ways of the old country, preferably an Italian speaker. Giuseppe—or George, as he called himself—the Boston son, was the only offspring with a suitable wife. George and his wife, Maria, owned a prosperous landscaping business in an affluent suburb. They lived in a spacious home that had just recently been vacated by their daughter, who had stayed with her parents until her marriage at age twenty-two. This development fortuitously provided a bedroom that could be redecorated for Angelina.

Angelina spent the next few years in her suburban American abode, busying herself with household chores, tending Maria's vegetable garden, acquiring a smattering of English, and qualifying for Medicare. On her seventy-fifth birthday, tipsy after drinking a few glasses of wine, she fell down the stairs, fracturing her skull and bleeding into her brain. In the eyes of her physicians, she made a remarkable recovery. To her family, she went from being entirely independent to needing help with bathing, dressing, and even eating. Salvatore tried to decree that his mother be cared for at home, but Maria, her primary caregiver, had just learned she had breast cancer and was undergoing chemotherapy. Giancarlo was between wives again. Luigi lived in a third-floor New York walk-up that was clearly inadequate. Salvatore himself lived in Chicago, which he argued would constitute too much of an upheaval for his mother. So Angelina Nicolazzo entered Golden Acres Nursing Home, her room and board paid for by Salvatore the investment banker. She did not have Alzheimer's disease, but her cognitive function had never returned to normal after her tumble.

Salvatore was a generous man and a devoted son, but the difference in cost between a semiprivate room and a private room was thirty dollars a day, or just under $11,000 a year. Salvatore's business success derived from a certain degree of conservatism, enhanced by flashes of intuition. He felt a similar strategy was appropriate in the care of his mother, who after all might easily live another ten years. The marginal cost of a private room for the next decade was over $100,000, which his business sense told him was extravagant. Since his siblings were most impressed by their oldest brother's calculations and conclusions, Angelina Nicolazzo was admitted to a double room, which she shared with Sylvia Truman.

For the first few weeks of their cohabitation, the two women barely conversed. But when Angelina, whose English had never been fluent and who tended increasingly to revert to Italian, discovered that Sylvia understood a little Italian, she was ecstatic. Sylvia had scarcely spoken Italian since childhood and proved to have as much word-finding difficulty in Italian as she did in English. So Sylvia spoke to Angelina in short English phrases and Angelina spoke to Sylvia in bursts of Italian. They often did not understand enough to respond appropriately, but they took comfort in each other's presence. After two months they became inseparable: they ate meals together, they attended activities jointly, and they wandered the circular corridor in tandem.

John Truman was delighted by his mother's roommate. Even though he did not speak more than a smattering of Italian and could understand very little of what Angelina said, he recognized her dedication to his mother. He particularly appreciated her neatness and her quietness. He saw how reassuring it was to Sylvia to share her life with a compatriot, with a woman whose roots, customs, culinary preferences, and native language were the same as hers. When John visited his mother, only to discover that her roommate had been hospitalized with a massive stroke that left her unable to swallow and had returned to the nursing home with a feeding tube, he was stunned and horrified.

"Is she comatose?" I asked, trying to grasp the medical facts.

"No, no. Her eyes open and she looks around. She follows people with her eyes. I'm not sure whether she recognizes anyone. She certainly didn't know me, and she didn't light up when she saw Mom, the way she used to."

"Can she speak at all?"

"She's totally paralyzed on her right side, and she can't say more than a few words—all Italian. She says 'Mama' a lot. Pretty much the only thing she does is to push away things she doesn't want."

"And is your mother very upset by all this?" I thought perhaps he felt Sylvia needed a tranquilizer.

"She is and she isn't. Most of the time I don't think she realizes the woman in the next bed is her friend Angelina. Maybe I'm imagining it, but sometimes I think she looks at her and shudders. Not because she misses Angelina, but because she doesn't want to be like that." I thought it highly unlikely that Sylvia had the capacity to imagine herself similarly impaired, but I remained silent and let John continue. "I suppose I'm just projecting. *I* shudder at the idea of my mother being like that. Not just paralyzed and unable to speak, though that's bad enough. But getting nutrition dripped into her through a tube connected to her stomach."

"What is it you find so distressing?" I pressed him for clarification.

"It's that Angelina is being kept alive when she has no *relationships* anymore. She's breathing and her heart's beating, so she isn't *dead*. But she doesn't seem like a person anymore. Before the stroke, she had lost a lot, and I guess her quality of life wasn't very good, but she was clearly a person. Just like Mom's a person, although very limited in her capacities. Mom can still have a relationship with another human being. She and Angelina were friends in their own way. If Mom ever had as devastating an illness as Angelina and could no longer swallow, I wouldn't want her to have a tube to feed her."

"That's fine," I responded quietly. "She wouldn't have to have one."

"If she could eat, of course, I wouldn't want her to starve." I didn't know if he was talking about Angelina or his mother, but suspected they were coalescing in his mind. "But that tube, with the white liquid flowing in—that's not *food*. Getting nourishment through a tube is no more like eating than"—he thought for a moment—"than artificial insemination is like sex." He laughed, but I knew he was deadly serious.

"You're right," I acknowledged. "There's a great deal of emotion attached to nutrition and hydration. But what people really want is for their relative to be cared for, to be kept comfortable. That means being kept clean, having their lips moistened, being turned from side to side, given oxygen for shortness of breath and morphine if needed for pain." I didn't want to deliver a lecture, but many people associate death by dehydration or starvation with concentration camps. By contrast, there is nothing to suggest that dying, comatose, or minimally responsive patients suffer if they are not artificially nourished or hydrated. Terminally ill cancer patients who are alert enough to describe their feelings typically do not report thirst or hunger when they lose the capacity to eat and drink.[4] From an ethical point of view, administration of intravenous solutions and tube feeding is not required to promote the patient's comfort. From a medical point of view, artificial hydration is ineffective in reversing the underlying pathology in an individual who is dying, although it may stave off death for a brief period. From a legal point of view, substances delivered by vein or by stomach tube are medical treatments, whether they are antibiotics, hormones, water, or protein. Patients or their surrogates may therefore refuse them just as they are entitled to decline any medical intervention.[5]

John Truman, struggling to maintain his equanimity at the other end of the line, knew all about the court cases. He wanted to guarantee that his mother would not suffer when the end came, and also to ensure that her dying would not be needlessly prolonged if she crossed the line between being a person with emotions and thoughts to being a mere organism. I assured him I would do my best to maximize Sylvia's comfort if she became acutely ill, and that I would discuss with him any proposed treatments so that we could together weigh the risks and benefits. "No machines," John stated. "Not even short-term."

"And no feeding tubes," I added.

"No feeding tubes," John concurred.

* * *

It was eleven at night when my beeper went off. I had learned to recognize its insistent cries for what they were: a call for help from a patient in distress. I fumbled for my glasses and pressed the button on the beeper, which simultaneously stilled its voice and caused a series of digits to be flashed on its miniature display screen. I recognized at once the telephone number of the Golden Acres Nursing Home.

Being on call was a responsibility I shared with three other doctors. In exchange for three weeks of peaceful evenings and undisturbed weekends, we each had one week when we were at risk of receiving calls from patients in the practices of any of the group's members. The two geriatricians in the group tended to have the sickest patients. In addition to our community-dwelling patients, we also cared for nursing home residents. The nurses in the nursing homes were required to notify a physician if a patient fell—even if he sustained no discernible injury—and to report any abnormal laboratory test results (which they never seemed to learn about before eight in the evening).

This was my week on call. It was only Thursday, but I was already tired from nightly disruptions of my sleep. I really could not complain, for I only seldom had to go to the hospital in the middle of the night. The hospital with which I was affiliated had house staff (interns and residents) on site at all times. They were fresh out of medical school—young and relatively inexperienced, but also energetic and immersed in the routines of acute care medicine. Some of the calls were from the emergency room, which was staffed by senior physicians as well as house officers, to let me know about a patient and to give me the opportunity to discuss the appropriate initial diagnostic evaluation and management. Other calls were from patients at home who needed advice: recommendations to go to the emergency room or to call their physician in the morning, advice to try milk of magnesia for constipation. Still other calls, like this one, were from the night nurse at a nursing home, requesting instructions on what to do about a resident who had become ill.

I had been impressed by Golden Acres by day, but nighttime was a different story. The night nurses were often less

well-trained, their English barely up to the task of communi-
cating their observations or of understanding my questions.
To add to the frustrations of night call, it was several minutes
before I was connected to the right floor. I had been paged
to the main number of the home, without any extension, and
of course the operator had no idea which nurse had called me.
By this time I had patients living on three different corridors
of Golden Acres, so I did not know who wanted me either. The
operator preferred not to use the overhead paging system at
night, for fear of awakening the residents, so she had no alternative but to call each nursing station in turn to inquire if they
had paged me. Since only one nurse was on duty on each floor
for the eleven to seven shift, and she was typically checking on
her patients, the telephone often rang for a long while before
anyone answered. I was on hold for six minutes before the
nurse who wanted to speak with me was located.

"I have a resident here who doesn't look so good." An ominous, if not altogether enlightening beginning.

"What's her name?" I asked.

"Sylvia Truman."

"In what way does she not look right?"

"She's breathing fast."

"How fast?" Respiratory rate is well correlated with the
severity of many illnesses and is a readily measurable quantity,
requiring only eyes, ears, and a watch with a second hand.

"About thirty a minute."

"Does she have a fever?"

"Yes, her temperature's a hundred one."

"What's her blood pressure?" Patients with a severe infection or profound dehydration accompanying their illness usually have low blood pressure.

"It's one twenty over eighty." That was a good sign. If the
systolic pressure, the top number, was one hundred or less,
then Sylvia would need immediate attention and intravenous
fluids if she was to have any chance of successful treatment.

I still did not know whether Sylvia's problem was primarily
respiratory. Just because she was breathing rapidly did not
mean she had a pulmonary illness—people breathe fast from
a fever alone, or to compensate for excessive acid in their
blood, or because of pain or anxiety. Patients with urosepsis—
bacteria from the bladder that had made their way into the

bloodstream—often look this way. I tried to gather a little more information. "Does she have any other symptoms? Does she have diarrhea? Is she vomiting? Does she have a cough?"

"She was coughing earlier. The nurse from the evening shift said she coughed during dinner."

Now that was a very useful clue. Many individuals with dementia, much like Sylvia's roommate who had had a stroke, lose their capacity to swallow reliably. They tend to aspirate food or saliva, whose usual complement of bacteria makes its way into the lungs when they eat, causing inflammation and then pneumonia.

My mind raced. I had to make a decision instantly. The nurse had thirty patients to attend to—she could not afford to spend any more time on the telephone. I could send Sylvia to the hospital, where she would spend the next three hours in the emergency room, maybe longer if it was busy. She would have a physical examination and chest X ray (potentially diagnostic of pneumonia), blood tests (to determine if she had an elevated white blood cell count, consistent with infection), a blood gas (a sample drawn from an artery to determine if she had sufficient oxygen in her blood). She would probably have a battery of other tests, too: an electrocardiogram (even if she unambiguously proved to have a pneumonia, the increased demand on her heart from a severe infection could overwhelm the heart, precipitating a heart attack) and a urinalysis (just in case she had a urinary tract infection, too). Odds were that at some point around three or four in the morning the decision would be made to admit her to the hospital. She would be moved from the highly uncomfortable stretcher where she had spent most of the night to an only marginally more comfortable hospital bed. She would then have her vital signs taken once again, this time by the nurse on the floor and, if she was lucky, she would drift off to sleep. Her sleep would be brief, however, as she would soon be due for a dose of intravenous antibiotics. Her nurse would switch on the light, waking her up again, so she could hook up the bag with the antibiotics to the plastic catheter in Sylvia's arm.

Alternatively, I could get dressed, drive out to Golden Acres, and have a look at Sylvia, without the benefit of technology beyond my stethoscope. If I decided she seemed very sick, I could send her to the hospital at what would then be after midnight. If I concluded that she most likely had a respiratory infection, whether bronchitis or the more dangerous pneumonia, but her illness appeared sufficiently mild that she could readily be treated with oral antibiotics, then I could order medication for her to receive at the nursing home.

Or I could decide based on what I had heard on the telephone that Sylvia Truman had aspirated at suppertime but was only moderately ill thus far. I could order oxygen for her breathing, Tylenol to lower her fever, antibiotics by mouth to combat the infection, and both Sylvia and I could go to sleep.

I was not a disinterested party to this decision. Driving to the nursing home in the middle of the night was distinctly unappealing. Even the emergency room route would be disruptive to me, as I would be in telephone contact with the emergency room physicians at least twice: once at the beginning of their assessment and once at the end of their evaluation. But I had to try to be objective, to do what was best for Sylvia Truman.

What shaped my decision was the conversation I had recently had with her son, John, in which he had articulated a course of action for just such a situation: he wanted tests and treatments only if they were not intrusive or painful. The goal of care was first of all Sylvia's comfort and only secondarily cure. Under the circumstances, I translated his directive to mean that Sylvia should not be sent to the hospital in the middle of the night to be scanned and bled, her bladder instrumented, and her heart recorded. She should be treated on site, in her own bed, for what was the most *likely* diagnosis rather than for a radiologically or bacteriologically *confirmed* disease. If the less intensive treatment available in the nursing home proved inadequate to cure her—either because the blood levels of the antibiotics achievable with pills were insufficient to combat the germs responsible for her infection, or because she in fact had a different disease that only the more thorough hospital procedure would have diagnosed—John would be sad but, I believed, not dissatisfied. She would have been spared the indignities of a hospitalization that, at best, could have returned her to her previous demented state and permitted her to become subsequently more demented or to develop another pneumonia. At worst, she would have become delirious, as she had after her hip fracture, or come down with yet another complication of hospitalization, or ended up even less functional after her infection was cured than she had been before it developed.[6]

I persuaded myself that the only reason to go to the nursing home was to determine if Sylvia was sick enough to justify hospitalization, and having concluded that she should not be hospitalized even if she qualified in a technical sense, there seemed little point to making the journey. I therefore requested that the nurse administer oxygen through a face mask, that she give Sylvia Tylenol every four hours, and that she start her on an antibiotic recommended for use in mild pneumonia. The nurse was satisfied. I went to bed.

It took a long time for me to fall asleep. Gone were the days of my internship, when I could fall asleep anywhere, anytime, when I could instantly shut off the jets of adrenaline turned on in moments of crisis. My mind was spinning. I reviewed the facts of Sylvia's case, to the extent that I knew them, over and over, searching for some critical omission, some other observation that would make a difference. When I had satisfied myself that I had chosen a reasonable course of action, I was still wide awake. I began thinking about all the things I needed to do the next day. I organized, planned, and then revised my plans. Well after midnight, I fell asleep.

The next morning, suffering from the predictable effect of insufficient sleep, I was grumpy. I perceived all my usual morning chores as an imposition: preparing my children's lunches, making the beds, driving my boys to school. When I reached my office at 8:30, I regarded the morning's roster of patients as yet another burden. But once I fell into the routine, my mood improved. Jeannette Schmidt was delighted to learn that her cough might be due to the blood pressure medication she had recently started taking, rather than anything more ominous. Melanie Jacobson was happy to get a flu shot. Donald Ryman and his son were pleased to hear that the memory deficit I had identified on an earlier visit was not appreciably worse.

Between patients, or while my patients were getting undressed, I responded to telephone messages. There was one from Golden Acres: Sylvia Truman was not any better. She was still febrile with a rapid respiratory rate. I ordered a blood test and a chest X ray—an outside lab was under contract to come in and provide these services during the day. A trip to the hospital to obtain these tests was necessary only at night. I did not expect that two doses of antibiotics would have brought the temperature down even if Sylvia did have pneumonia, but I had hoped that with the oxygen and the Tylenol she would at least be more comfortable. Her heart rate was up, reflecting her continuing distress, which was not a good sign.

By midafternoon I received the test results: "Poor inspiratory effort. Underpenetrated film. Increased markings at the bases consistent with probably bilateral infiltrates. No effusions or congestive heart failure." In other words, the radiologist reading the film could not be certain, but Sylvia probably had pneumonia involving the lower lobes of both lungs. The white blood cell count was reported at about the same time: another technician, from another lab, had drawn a tube of blood and brought the precious specimen to a large commercial laboratory, together with samples from a half dozen other residents whose physicians had ordered a blood sugar or thyroid functions. The white cell count was 18,000, markedly elevated, with a disproportionate number of infection-fighting cells, strongly suggesting the presence of alien bacteria somewhere in the body.

It was Friday afternoon, with a weekend looming. I decided I had better have a look at Sylvia Truman myself. My planned trip to the library would have to be postponed again. I headed out to suburban Golden Acres before rush hour traffic built up.

Sylvia was lying in bed, perspiring, working hard to breathe. Her eyes were open but all she said when I addressed her was "I, I, I." I adjusted the oxygen mask, which she had pushed off her nose and mouth and which was aerating her forehead instead. I tried listening to her chest, but she would not follow my instructions to take deep breaths with her mouth open any more than she had heeded the X-ray technician, so my exam was similarly limited. I satisfied myself that she was not wheezing, which could have meant that asthma medication would help, and that she did not have fluid in her lungs from a failing heart. Her blood pressure was excellent, and her lips did not have the dusky blue tinge of a person with a dangerously low oxygen level. The nurse assured me that although Sylvia had not touched her food, she had had plenty to drink.

I wrote a note in Sylvia's chart, continued the oxygen and antibiotics, exhorted the staff to ply Sylvia with fluids so she would not become dehydrated, left a message on John Truman's answering machine to update him, and went back to the office.

When I returned to work after the weekend, I half expected to find Sylvia in the hospital, despite my emphasizing to the covering doctor that the overriding goal of care was comfort. No, the computer did not show Sylvia Truman as an impatient in the hospital. She might not have made it through the weekend. I spoke with my colleague about other admissions, phone calls, discharges. He had not heard from Golden Acres. Evidently, Sylvia's temperature had come down, her breathing had eased, and she was on the mend.

My next monthly visit to Golden Acres was brief. The former teacher, Annette Simonson, was experiencing uncontrollable crying jags. She was unable to say what was upsetting her. A well-meaning arm around her shoulders just made her cry harder. Milton and Mildred Schwartz, the husband and wife, had been quarreling. They would yell at each other, and when a nurse tried to intercede, they could not remember what they had been fighting about. The following day they did not remember the altercation had taken place. Unless their volatility escalated into a regular occurrence, I was reluctant to medicate either of them.

The high point of the visit took place when I saw a relatively new patient, Margaret Coughlin. Mrs. Coughlin was a physically vigorous woman in her eighties whose dementia had left her markedly less self-conscious than in her younger days. Her dementia affected the frontal lobes of the brain, producing disinhibition and apathy. In some people, this leads to socially inappropriate behavior such as public displays of sexuality or disrobing. Margaret was simply far more relaxed than she had been previously. She said whatever was on her mind, whether it was "Gee, that nurse has a big rear end" or "It really stinks in here." As a younger woman she had gone through three husbands, none of whom could live up to her high standards and finicky demands. Her daughters reported that she had been chronically miserable—and had made their lives miserable when they were growing up. She had never been satisfied with them. She had always complained and never complimented, violating the basic tenet of every book on parenting, with predictable consequences: her daughters were insecure, were forever searching for approval, and despised her. They started out visiting the nursing home out of filial obligation rather than out of love. But over time, as their mother became more accepting of them, they came to see a new side of her. She was funny. Witty comments about everyone around her replaced her earlier hypercritical remarks. She made amusing observations that others would be too embarrassed to state aloud.

Mrs. Coughlin was also considerably happier than she had been before she developed dementia. She no longer worried about her blood pressure—she simply took the medication the nurses gave her. As a result, her average blood pressure was significantly lower than it had been earlier in her life. She had no doubt been a victim of "white coat hypertension," or elevations in pressure far more marked when she was tested in the doctor's office than when she tested herself at home with her own blood pressure cuff. Margaret was similarly much less nervous about her arthritis than she had been when she lived at home. At one time, she worried that every twinge presaged total disability and dependence. She imagined that she would be unable to write and that she would be in pain every day. Her worst fear—one she had dwelled on, telephoning her daughters in a panic at frequent intervals—was that she would spend the rest of her life in a wheelchair. Now, she notified the nurse if her joints hurt, and if they still bothered her by the time the nurse came back with a Tylenol, she took one; if she had forgotten about the arthritis, she cheerfully waved the nurse away and suggested she give the pill to the man across the hall, who, she observed, looked like he had a headache.

When I paid my respects to Margaret Coughlin that chilly November day, she smiled at me as though we were old friends. "How are you?" she asked, with genuine warmth.

"I'm fine," I replied and then asked, suspecting that she mistook me for someone else, "Do you remember me?"

"Sure!" she laughed. "You're the lady who runs the bingo."

"Actually," I answered matter-of-factly, "I'm your doctor."

"Oh." Margaret frowned, looking puzzled. "Are you sure?"

"Quite sure. That is, if you're Margaret Coughlin."

"That's me! Have we met before?" I told her we had, but it had been some time ago (one month, to be exact, since state regulations mandated monthly visits to nursing home residents).

"Now I remember!" she exclaimed, after looking me over intently. "Your hair was shorter last time." I had not had a haircut in the interim, so my hair probably had been an inch shorter on my prior visit. "You should have it cut," she recommended. "You won't find a husband if you don't worry about your looks." I informed her goodnaturedly that I appreciated her advice, but I was already married.

"Really!" She was amazed. I told her that not only was I married, but I also had three sons.

"Can't be!" She spoke in exclamations. "You're too young to have three children." I had noticed that to many of my patients who were over eighty, everyone under fifty seemed youthful. In Margaret Coughlin's case, her judgment was impaired due to her dementia, and she tended to say whatever popped into her mind, so I was not surprised that she had no sense of my age. I assured her that I was quite old enough to have children—and to be her doctor.

"Three, though, that's a handful. Boys? Girls?" Usually I do not like to divulge much about my personal life to my patients, but the basic demographics were fair game, and I was learning about Margaret's cognitive function as we spoke. Her language was quite good, though her sentences were very short. Her memory was clearly poor, and she tended to confabulate—to make up answers to questions to cover up for her deficiencies, as when she said she knew me. It might have been a simple case of mistaken identity, but when I tested her by asking whether I had seen her in the supermarket earlier in the week, she beamed and told me how I had been buying popcorn for my sons. This kind of confabulation is a classic feature of alcoholic dementia, but people with other forms of dementia use the same strategy in a vain effort to compensate for their inadequacies.

I asked Margaret how she was feeling, concluded that she was thriving at Golden Acres (in fact she had gained ten pounds over the three months since her admission), and moved on to Sylvia Truman.

Sylvia had never regained her baseline level of function after the pneumonia. She had remained delirious—confused and agitated—for two weeks after her fever had come down and her cough had subsided. During that entire period, she had emerged from her room only for meals, spending most of the day in a chair but retreating to her room for both a morning and an afternoon nap. When she was finally cured of her pneumonia, she remained physically weak. Any illness in a physically frail or demented older person can produce the same debilitating effect. Pneumonia, once called the old man's friend by William Osler, the medical luminary of the turn of the century, today kills its victims in only a minority of cases. But its capacity to cause weakness and confusion is undiminished.

When I arrived on C corridor, Sylvia was sitting in a wheel-chair, staring vacantly in front of her, her hands folded in her lap as usual. I said hello, and she greeted me politely, as she would any stranger. I shook her hand and noticed she was slightly stiff, almost like a person with Parkinson's disease. In the later stages of Alzheimer's disease, individuals frequently develop rigidity. Their faces show little expression, although in the patients with Parkinson's, there may be feelings hidden behind the immobile face, whereas in the Alzheimer's patient, the blank face often reflects an emotionless reality.

I asked Sylvia to get up out of her seat, but her arm muscles were so wasted that she could not propel herself from her chair, even when she leaned on the armrests. Once I helped her up, she was very unsteady. I held onto her as she took a few shuffling steps, but then nearly fell backward. I eased her back into her chair. Clearly she could no longer walk without considerable assistance. Her gait disorder was probably multi-factorial, as were so many geriatric disturbances. The quadri-ceps, the big muscles of the thighs, were weak, atrophied from weeks of disuse. The rigidity I had detected in her arms affected her legs as well. Her judgment, which enabled her to figure out what to do if she encountered an obstacle, was impaired. And her vision was declining. She had cataracts in both eyes. Her visual deficit was still mild—she could recognize her son halfway across the room and she was able to watch television—but it was probably sufficient to contribute to her hesitancy as she walked.

I checked Sylvia's lungs to find out if she had any residual changes after the bout of pneumonia—she did not—and wrote a brief note in her chart: "Lungs clear. Recovered from pneumonia but strikingly weak. Unable to stand unassisted. Rigid but without tremor or bradykinesia to suggest Parkinson's. Findings consistent with advanced Alzheimer's disease. Overriding goal of treatment is supportive." I was not sure whether John would even want antibiotics administered if Sylvia again developed pneumonia.

The head nurse was shocked when I mentioned that John might have second thoughts about as seemingly innocuous a treatment as oral medication. "But we couldn't fail to treat her. That would be killing her!"

I told her about a special unit for severely demented patients at a local Veterans Administration Hospital whose philosophy was to offer hospice care. Families or officially appointed health care proxies are asked to select one of four possible approaches to care: maximal care (all potentially indicated treatment) at one extreme, palliative care (interventions intended exclusively to promote comfort, such as oxygen or pain medication), at the other extreme, and varying levels of aggressiveness in between.[7] A full 63 percent select palliative care, with the majority of the remaining families opting for the second, or marginally more extensive style of care. This level encompasses all intervention available at the nursing home, which in practical terms means blood tests, urine tests, chest X rays, and oral medication.

The nurse was intrigued by the existence of such an institution. She was surprised when I told her that a study of the outcomes of the residents in that unit showed that patients with fever who were treated with antibiotics did not fare any better than those who were not. In part this unexpected finding arose because many of the patients were so debilitated that they were likely to die from a bacterial infection, whether they received antibiotics or not: medication to kill germs was clearly only one ingredient of cure. In part, the similarity in outcomes reflected the fact that many febrile patients probably had self-limited, viral infections, which typically resolved without treatment. Sylvia's nurse listened with interest.

* * *

I anticipated that Sylvia would again develop pneumonia, since aspiration was usually a recurrent problem in demented individuals once they developed difficulty swallowing. After that single episode, she never developed a full-blown pneumonia. But the day came when Sylvia no longer knew what to do with the food that was spooned into her mouth. Sometimes she pocketed it—chewing for a while and then squirreling the masticated wad in her cheek. Sometimes she seemed to play with it, sliding a morsel from side to side, but then spitting it out, like chewing gum that has lost its flavor. When she did swallow her food, she often coughed and choked on it. Sylvia's total intake of food fell far below the minimum necessary to sustain her, and she began losing weight.

At Golden Acres, Sylvia received most of her care from a nursing assistant named Gwen Gabriel. Gwen cared for five women and two men much like Sylvia in their level of function. She treated each of them as an individual: she knew, for example, that Sylvia preferred dresses to slacks. At one time, Sylvia Truman could argue vociferously that it was undignified for women to wear pants. She quoted from the Bible that "a woman must not put on man's apparel . . . for whoever does these things is abhorrent to the Lord your God."[8] She no longer knew *why* she preferred dresses, but she had imprinted in the surviving parts of her memory strong negative associations with pants. Gwen also knew from the photographs of Sylvia with her family that adorned her room how she had always worn her hair. Gwen brushed and combed Sylvia's hair to emulate the style in the pictures, and reminded the nursing staff to schedule an appointment at the beauty parlor whenever her hair started to become unmanageably long. If she had the time, Gwen polished Sylvia's nails, because Marcia had told her that her mother's major vanity was painting her nails. Gwen liked putting a little rouge on her charges. Sylvia seldom went outside and had the pale, drawn face of a shut-in—one who wasn't eating well or exercising either. With a dash of blush on her cheeks, she looked livelier, healthier.

Gwen took pride in her work. She was a deeply religious woman who had the gift of seeing the spark of humanity in

each of the patients she cared for. Their relationship was inti-
mate, as Gwen dressed and toileted all of them. She bathed
the women, but a special "bath orderly" showered the men.
Gwen brought all seven into the dining room at mealtimes.
Two could eat independently, three could manage on their
own once their food was cut up, and two, including Sylvia,
needed to be fed.

Mealtimes were becoming longer and more arduous. There
were days when Sylvia refused to open her mouth. There were
times when she pushed the spoon away and, if Gwen persisted
in trying to feed her, she gave her faithful attendant's arm
a surprisingly forceful shove. Gwen was persistent. She regarded Sylvia's rejection of food as a personal failure. She
tried giving Sylvia a fifteen-minute break and then once again
began coaxing her to eat. She tried waiting until all the other
residents had left the room so Sylvia would not be distracted.
Gwen even brought in a special rice pudding she baked herself. She tried nutritional supplements—drinks like Sustacal
or Ensure—between meals. Nothing worked.

The staff called a family meeting. John and Marcia came.
The floor nurse, the nursing home social worker, Gwen, and I
all attended. The issue of artificial feeding—of a gastrostomy
tube—had come up when Angelina had had a stroke. At that
time John had been firm: no feeding tubes. But now the discussion was not theoretical: we were not talking about
another person or what we would do if Sylvia ever got to the
point where she could not be nourished by mouth. We were
talking about Sylvia and we were talking about the present.
There were two choices: to continue to try to feed her, knowing that her intake was insufficient and that what she did take
in might well end up in her lungs instead of her stomach, or
we could insert a tube for feeding directly through the
abdominal wall into the stomach.

John wanted to know just what "G-tube placement" involved. I told him it required an operation, though a relatively minor one. Sylvia would be hospitalized. While under
anesthesia, an endoscope would be passed from her mouth to
her stomach to allow the surgeon to see what he was doing.
Then an incision would be made in the skin overlying the
abdomen so that a rubber tube could be inserted into the
stomach (a gastrostomy tube) or into the small intestine (a

jejunostomy tube). Looking through the endoscope, the surgeon could secure the rubber tube. Then he would remove the endoscope, and in a day or two the nurses could pump Sustacal directly into the intestinal tract.

I had never seen John so stern and remote. He had always been affable and approachable. "What are the risks?" he asked, businesslike.

"The usual risk of anesthesia. A small chance of perforating an organ. Transient increase in confusion after the procedure."

John's sense of humor prevailed. "How would you know if she's *more* confused? Do you have some sort of meter to measure that? I didn't think anyone could get more confused."

I corrected myself. "She could become temporarily agitated, much as she did after she broke her hip."

"That's it?"

"Well, the problem is not so much the procedure itself, though that's not totally risk free, but later on. Often people pull out the tube and it has to be reinserted. That's not a tremendous ordeal—a new tube can be put in at the bedside without anesthesia or endoscopy. Still, it's a nuisance. People who repeatedly pull out their G-tubes usually end up having their hands restrained so they won't do it anymore." John flinched. "Moreover, while a G-tube can guarantee that Sylvia gets adequate nutrition, it doesn't prevent aspiration. The stuff that's dripped in can still back up the tube and make its way to the lungs."

Marcia looked puzzled. "Even though she wouldn't be eating the normal way, she could still develop pneumonia?" I nodded.

"How diabolical," John muttered.

"And finally, one of my colleagues recently did a study that showed that patients with advanced dementia who have G-tubes put in to feed them live no longer than comparable patients without tubes."[9] I let that sink in.

John and Marcia looked at each other with that perfect, soundless communication that is occasionally possible between siblings.

"No feeding tubes," John stated. The meeting was over.

Sylvia dwindled rapidly. She lost a great deal of weight in the next few weeks. She never said she had any pain, and she showed no evidence through her facial expressions of being in pain. She did not throw up or have trouble breathing, both common occurrences in dying patients.[10] Sylvia became progressively weaker until one day she stopped eating. She could not explain why—did she feel as though food was getting stuck on the way down, which would suggest a cancer of the esophagus? Did food trigger abdominal pain, perhaps indicative of a stomach malignancy? Sylvia could not explain herself, but she unambiguously pushed away the hand that sought to feed her. She refused breakfast and lunch, and again would not eat at dinner. The following day she would not drink either. She was so weak that the nurses kept her in bed. In another day she was barely arousable—she would open her eyes if her name was called repeatedly, only to close them again if she was not continually stimulated. One more day and she no longer opened her eyes at all. Her pulse remained strong and her breathing was unlabored.

Five days after she stopped eating and drinking, Sylvia Truman's blood pressure began to drop. Her legs became mottled from poor perfusion. Her respirations became shallow. Her heart rate was irregular. Sylvia's nurse called the family to notify them that the end was imminent. John, Cynthia, and Marcia all rushed over to Golden Acres. They sat by Sylvia's bedside, awkward, unsure what to do or say because she seemed oblivious to their presence. They were afraid to leave for dinner, lest she die while they were all out of the room. Finally, after several hours during which she was unchanged, they agreed to take turns going out. At eleven at night they asked the nurse how long Sylvia could go on like this, barely alive. She told them that it could not be much longer. They felt guilty, waiting for her to die. All three of them remained in her room and one after another dozed off in their chairs.

Cynthia woke up at five in the morning to go to the bathroom. When she returned, the room seemed eerily quiet. She realized that her mother-in-law's slow, noisy breathing had stopped. She let out a cry, awakening John and Marcia. They turned on the light and found Sylvia absolutely still, her mouth open, the same empty expression on her face that she had exhibited in the last months of her life. John went to

fetch the nurse and the nurse called me to come and "pro-
nounce" Sylvia.

I stopped at the nursing home on my way to work to certify
officially that Sylvia Truman had died, and to fill out the
death certificate. Her family were all still there, simultaneously sad, exhausted, and relieved. I told them what a great
family they were, how wonderful they had been to Sylvia. We
shook hands and said good-bye.

There was a void in me all day, partly because death is
always draining, even a death that is welcomed and expected.
But Sylvia had been gone a long time: as far as I was concerned, she had started to separate from the world when she
moved to the nursing home. She had started to fade away
after her roommate's stroke, following which she never again
formed a relationship with another person. She had ceased
recognizing me months earlier, and only questionably knew
her family. But as Sylvia had become increasingly withdrawn
and uncommunicative, her son's role in deciding on her care
had become correspondingly greater. He had always been an
active participant in medical decision making, but over time
he had become his mother's voice. Now she was gone, and I
would no longer have any contact with the Trumans. I had
already said farewell to Sylvia, but John's grin and good-
natured way of dealing with his mother, Cynthia's nervous
devotion, and Marcia's deep love, which had made it so hard
for her to face her mother's decline, would all linger in my
memory. I would miss all of them.

Epilogue

When I began writing this book, I did so out of a passionate conviction that Alzheimer's disease was so awful that every able-minded American should be alerted to its horrors. I shared fully the views skillfully propagated by lay advocacy groups that Alzheimer's disease is the "disease of the century" that "steals the mind" and is like "a funeral that never ends." Above all, it is a "silent epidemic" to which the general public, despite increasing media attention over the last twenty years, is still largely indifferent.

Even with the publicity surrounding Alzheimer's disease after Ronald Reagan's diagnosis, I was convinced that Americans just did not grasp the awfulness of this disease. The coverage stimulated by Reagan's bittersweet letter to the American people revealing his condition was, I had to admit, accurate and comprehensive. The statistics were all there; the descriptions of the pathology, the course of the disease, the lack of treatment were all there. Yet I remained convinced that most people would regard Reagan's misfortune as a rarity, an unusual disease that was unlikely to strike *them*. Perhaps because of the concerted effort by the gerontologic establishment to recast old age as a time of continued growth and possibility rather than as a period of decline and decay, I was afraid that the importance of Alzheimer's disease as the "gray plague" would be underestimated. The admirable attempt to persuade the public of the "myth of senility" might, I worried, have been *too* successful: reassured that old people could think and behave much as had their younger selves, they would merely shake their heads pityingly at the sight of a person with Alzheimer's.[1] It seemed to me essential that every adult understand both that cognitive decline was not inevitable with age *and* that a very large proportion of the very old (those over eighty) *do* suffer from that process of relentless intellectual deterioration known as dementia.

I continue to believe that to achieve a deep understanding of Alzheimer's disease, we must feel the texture of the illness. To go further, to grasp the meaning of dementia in contemporary society, which in turn affects the nature of the experience for those with the disease, we have to examine the political, scientific, and historic underpinnings of the disease. Having vastly increased my own knowledge about these various aspects of dementia, subjects that are typically invisible to the clinician as well as to the general public, I am even more certain than I expected to be of the value of this material. Not only does the study of the historical and political background clarify how we see Alzheimer's disease and why; it also serves to illuminate the way American science works and how institutional forces conspire with intellectual trends to produce change.

Researching and writing this book have, however, subtly but powerfully altered my personal attitude to individuals with Alzheimer's disease. I still recoil when I imagine developing Alzheimer's myself or worry that those I love could be manifesting its symptoms. I still find taking care of large numbers of people with advanced dementia depressing and prefer not to have a clinical practice composed primarily of individuals with Alzheimer's. Having said all that, I nonetheless recognize what I failed to appreciate earlier: most individuals with mild to moderate dementia lead lives that are quite tolerable to them. They continue to have meaningful relationships with other people; they experience the full gamut of human emotions, from joy to despair; and their will to live remains very strong. This is not to deny that they may become depressed—roughly 40 to 50 percent of individuals with dementia become depressed at some point during the course of their illness. They may likewise feel frustrated by their inability to remember or to do things themselves, and at times exhibit anger when they are asked to accept help. But in most cases they adjust to their dependence, just as an individual with physical disabilities often adjusts to his condition.

Alzheimer's disease is different from other forms of disability, not merely because it involves the mind rather than the body, but because the particular way in which the mind is involved produces lack of insight into the disability. As observers, we may find the absence of awareness especially troubling, as though people would be able to resist their loss of cognitive function if only they knew what was happening to them. Our model of the noble way to respond to chronic disease is to fight, to struggle to maintain our independence, and through the process of resistance, to retain our dignity as human beings. Dementia, whose victims cannot grasp what hit them and whose only form of fighting is denial, does not fit our categories of ennobling diseases. From the point of view of the person with dementia, the failure to understand that one has a progressive brain disease may be the saving grace of the disorder. It allows that individual to enjoy his meals and the attention of his family, to sit peacefully tapping his foot to rhythmic songs on the radio, and to savor the excitement of soap operas on television.

Quality of life is more difficult to assess for those with advanced dementia—either the end-stage person who spends his time in bed or propped in a chair, or the slightly less end-stage person who paces and wanders incessantly. They have typically lost so much of their language function that they can communicate neither pleasure nor sadness. We can to a limited extent infer their emotions from their smiles and their grimaces, but with time their affect is increasingly blunted: they seem to experience very little. Any presumption, however, that the severely demented person is *suffering* by virtue of his very existence is a projection of our own dread at his condition. The old person with dementia whose limbs have stiffened and who groans when he is moved or washed is undoubtedly experiencing discomfort during those brief moments when things are done to him. To conclude, however, that he is miserable and would be better off dead is simply wrong: his current best interests (as opposed to any previously stated wishes about what he regarded as important or how he wished to be treated if he developed dementia) favor continued survival as long as he is still conscious. A person who enters what is technically known as a persistent vegetative state or coma, as occurs sometimes after head trauma or massive stroke, loses the last vestiges of personhood. The individual in the final stages of Alzheimer's disease has precious little personhood left, but he has some, and that small residual spark often responds to gentle voices or a soft touch or soothing melodies.[2]

Having said that people with dementia are often contented with their lot, or at least not overtly discontented, I do not mean to suggest that we should therefore do everything technically feasible to prolong their lives. The major reason that an aggressive medical strategy is undesirable, however, is not that the quality of life of those with dementia is poor. The overriding argument against invasive medical care is that the burdens of such treatment are almost certain to outweigh any benefits. The price of technologically sophisticated medical care is great because the uncomprehending demented person will likely need to be tied down and sedated in order to perform that CAT scan or that bone marrow biopsy, or even to receive intravenous medications. The price is steep because individuals with underlying "brain failure" (to coin a term comparable to respiratory failure or kidney failure or heart failure) is particularly prone to develop side effects from conventional medical therapy. Quite apart from the dangers and discomforts of being restrained, medications are risky in all old people and in all demented people and are doubly risky in old, demented people. Anesthesia and surgery, through a process that is far from completely understood, have a strong tendency to induce acute confusion in people with dementia—hallucinations and belligerence and disorientation over and beyond their baseline. The benefits of medical therapy, at best, are to restore the person to his prior state of impairment. No treatment for an acute medical problem is going to improve his underlying cognitive dysfunction. Given that the majority of severely demented individuals are also very old (usually well over eighty), their maximum life expectancy, if they are cured of their acute illness, is fairly short. Some octogenarians live to be ninety-five or one hundred, but typically they have at most a couple of years remaining. Putting together the risks of treatment and the limited potential benefits, maximal medical therapy for the demented makes sense only if you believe that any expense is justified if it increases even slightly the chance of survival.

Opting to forgo certain sorts of medical interventions does not imply disdaining *all* medical treatment. Rather, it is consistent with substituting intermediate care for maximal care whenever there is an alternative treatment offering reasonable prospects for success but only a low level of discomfort or risk. It means favoring home or nursing home care over hospital care, oral medications over intravenous medications, and medical treatment over surgical treatment. It starts with the assumption that the primary goal of medical treatment is not prolongation of life but rather maintenance of function (in those who retain certain functions such as walking or listening or observing) or maximization of comfort (in those whose only remaining functions are the most primitive ones such as breathing and swallowing).

My views about what constitutes appropriate medical treatment for those with dementing illness remain unchanged as I wind down my research. But the realization that a great many people with dementia are quite happy with their lives, or at least not abjectly miserable, leads me to believe that we as a society need to strive to modify our attitude toward the demented elderly. The prevailing view is that dementia is an unusual condition, afflicting only those who fail to take the necessary precautions, a disease not of paramount concern given its rarity and the likelihood that it will soon be curable. Those who do succumb to Alzheimer's disease—either because of bad genes or mental sloth—are a source of pity and dread. Instead, we should learn to acknowledge the reality that dementia is common among the old-old and that those who have it could have done nothing to prevent it. We need to accept people with cognitive impairment just as we are gradually coming to terms with people who have physical disabilities. The widespread claims that Alzheimer's disease destroys the personality and robs individuals of their minds ignore the fundamental truth that those with dementia are people with a disease. The disorder does not strip them of their humanity. Alzheimer's disease prevents people from doing many of the things they formerly did, many of the things that they previously valued highly, perhaps even the pursuits that defined them. They may no longer be exactly the same person they once were—though surely more closely related than anybody else—but with all their limitations, they are still people.

The humane response to an individual with dementia is compassionate acceptance, not disdain or disgust. I indicated earlier that our repugnance toward dementia stems in large part from the American passion for control—and dementia is, above all, a disease of loss of autonomy. The more I reflect on chronic illness generally, the more convinced I become that the prevailing way of thinking about *all* chronic disease is extremely unfortunate. Alzheimer's disease, with its effect on the capacity of for self-determination, represents the extreme of a more general problem.

The kinds of diseases we as a society (including physicians) are most comfortable with are acute and reversible. Bacterial infections such as pneumococcal pneumonia are the proto-types of the ideal disease: the patient suddenly develops symptoms, physical examination together with an X ray and perhaps a sputum test clinch the diagnosis, antibiotics are prescribed, and in ten days the patient is back to her usual activities. Diseases amenable to surgical cure are equally acceptable: gallstones that are treated by removal of the gall-bladder or breast cancer treated with excision of the offending part. Even a heart attack, which is really only the most dramatic manifestation of chronic atherosclerotic heart disease, appeals to modern sensibilities because it is custom-arily treated vigorously over a period of days. The treatment may entail blood-thinning medication, delivered by vein, as well as assorted drugs to improve the heart's pumping, or it may include a procedure such as angioplasty to physically push aside the material clogging the blood vessels that nourish the heart. In extreme situations treatment involves emergency bypass surgery. While the person who has had a heart attack may not be cured of his heart disease by his hos-pitalization, and the woman with breast cancer faces the pos-sibility of subsequent metastatic disease—and even the patient with pneumonia might develop repeated bouts of infection if he has an underlying pulmonary disease such as emphysema—the widespread perception is that the illness has resolved once the crisis is over. Moreover, the afflicted individual is assumed to be the same as he was previously, once he is "cured." What is very hard for us to come to terms with is an illness that can at best be ameliorated or controlled, but that lingers, following a relapsing and remitting course like the neurodegenerative disease multiple sclerosis, or the joint disease rheumatoid arthritis, or a relentlessly downhill course such as AIDS or pancreatic cancer.

The chronic illnesses all irrevocably change their hosts. They cannot so readily be seen as outside invaders, like bacteria or other infectious agents that enter the body, wreak havoc, are attacked—and hopefully repulsed. Some of the acute illnesses, of course, leave a certain amount of destruction in their wake. Their victims may not be precisely the same after the onslaught as before: meningitis, for example, an infection of the lining of the brain and spinal cord, even if cured, may cause residual hearing loss. Curative surgery may disfigure or produce loss of sensation in the skin overlying the operative site due to nerve damage. But if the acute illness leaves a scar behind, that deficit is typically stable; it is not something that gets worse over time, or that insidiously alters the affected individual. Chronic illnesses, by contrast, characteristically produce progressive changes. Legs gradually stop moving, vision fades over time, and joints stiffen and swell. The person with the illness is, in a fundamental way, changed.

Our tendency is to try to externalize chronic illness just as we do acute illness: "it" (the diabetes or the Parkinson's or the arthritis) has affected "my" legs or "my" eyes. "It" causes "me" to have trouble walking or seeing. A brain disease like Alzheimer's may, at first glance, appear to affect *me* directly—not merely some desirable but nonessential bodily part. Alzheimer's, one might think, strikes the one indispensable part, the seat of the person. In fact, a person with dementia, when she talks about her condition, says her memory "is not working right," or she "gets disoriented," or she cannot "do addition" anymore. But her sense of self is intact. Even when I ask a question of a demented patient whose language capacity is almost entirely lost, she will start to answer "I, I, I . . ." The notion that all chronic illnesses except dementia (and possibly psychiatric illness, which also affects the mind) leave the *essential* part of the person untouched, affecting only organs of peripheral importance, is sheer fantasy. Our bodily parts are not merely cogs in a machine, fully replaceable, transplant surgery notwithstanding. A person who has chronic renal failure necessitating dialysis is inevitably altered by his disease. This is both because he will have significant levels of various toxins circulating in his blood at various times, despite the thrice-weekly cleansing by the dialysis machine, and because the process of spending upwards of twelve hours a week hooked up to a machine is bound to leave a mark on him. Whether the consequence is to affect his sense of his own fragility or to make him angry at his misfortune or grateful that he is alive in the late twentieth century, the experience changes him. He may still be good-natured or funny or ill-humored, but because of the repeated and powerful confrontations with disease over a prolonged period, he will invariably be shaped by his illness. Disturbances in different parts of the body can be expected to have varying effects: severe psoriasis, a skin disease causing scaly plaques on much of the body, affects the appearance; rheumatoid arthritis, which often deforms and cripples the hands, interferes with the ability to manipulate the world; and Alzheimer's disease disturbs the capacity to think, reason, and remember. To argue that Alzheimer's is totally different from all other chronic diseases is to espouse a radical mind-body dualism. While some chronic diseases change people more drastically than others, and while no disease transforms an individual into a new person entirely, all chronic disorders leave their mark.

If I am right that chronic illness inevitably changes the person with the illness, then the appropriate response to being ill is to accept the changes. This does not mean that a woman paralyzed by a stroke should refuse the physical therapist's efforts to help her walk again, or that the man whose leg has been amputated should stoically deny himself a prosthesis. It does not mean that a woman with Alzheimer's disease should continue her habit of drinking wine with dinner or taking over-the-counter antihistamines for her allergies, both of which run the risk of exacerbating her confusion. There is a narrow line between *acceptance* and *resignation*. I think that striving to maximize one's function—whether walking or thinking—is an admirable goal. What does not make sense to me is to apply our standards and expectations for acute illness to chronic illness. Using the military lingo so commonly adopted in speaking of disease, we should not expect to "attack" the disease and "conquer" our disabilities. For if our goal is eradication of an enemy invader, we are destined to lose the battle.

Society expects that modern medicine can cure disease with a magic bullet or, failing that, eliminate suffering. Even the dying, who may have reached the point where they no longer anticipate a miracle cure, continue to demand complete relief from pain. Desperately ill indviduals have increasingly been demanding physician-assisted suicide in large measure because they believe they are entitled to the total abolition of suffering. The idea that suffering is part of the human condition, that physicians have an obligation to *ameliorate* pain but not necessarily to obliterate it, is alien to contemporary sensibilities.[3] Likewise, individuals with chronic illness need to accept themselves as they are. With Alzheimer's disease, paradoxically, patients often do accept their limitations, though at times they may also be anxious, fearful, or depressed. With dementing illness, the added challenge is for *families* and caregivers to acknowledge that Mom is still Mom despite her deficits. The cognitive dissonance engendered by the fact that Mom has changed but is still Mom sometimes leads to the conclusion that Mom is now another person altogether—and sometimes to the conclusion that she has not changed significantly at all, even when the objective reality strongly suggests otherwise.

Just because people with Alzheimer's disease need to accept their condition and be accepted by others does not imply a diminished role for lay advocacy groups. On the contrary, the mission of organizations such as the Alzheimer's Association to provide education, to stimulate public awareness, and to lobby for programs for afflicted persons is essential. Individuals with Alzheimer's have profited from the growth of adult day care programs and home care services that make it feasible to remain at home longer. They have benefited from the development of special care units and assisted living apartments when they can no longer remain at home. These caretaking arrangements have arisen from the political pressure exerted by advocacy groups—principally on government to enact legislation funding assistance programs used by those with Alzheimer's.

Nor does the need to come to terms with dementia imply that the scientific establishment's efforts to understand the cause and mechanism of Alzheimer's are of no consequence. If Alzheimer's disease can one day be prevented or cured, then it will go the way of tuberculosis—a chronic, usually fatal disease in the nineteenth century, which is a relatively rare and curable infectious disease in the Western world today.[4] The laboratories throughout the country that are working on elucidating the role of amyloid and the more recently discovered tau protein should continue their work with a vengeance. Competition among those labs serves as a stimulus to more and better research. If the National Institute on Aging continues to fund scientific research on Alzheimer's, and the genetic, biochemical, and physiological basis of the disease are unraveled at an ever-escalating pace, then one day a cure may be found. When that happens, this book will be obsolete, or at best of historical interest. I look forward to that day. In the meantime, the scientific work, fueled by politicking in the best sense of the word, should continue. And we all need to grapple with understanding the experience of having Alzheimer's disease because, until that day comes, we are all at risk.

Appendix: Resources and Recommended Reading

Self-Help Books

Cohen, Donna, and Eisdorfer, Carl. *The Loss of Self: A Family Resource for the Care of Alzheimer's Disease and Related Disorders.* New York: W. W. Norton, 1986. A self-help book written from a psychiatric perspective.

Harvard Health Letter. "A Special Report: Alzheimer's Disease." Boston: Harvard Medical School Health Publications Group, 1994. A carefully written summary of the science of Alzheimer's, written for a general audience.

Mace, Nancy, and Rabins, Peter. *The Thirty-Six Hour Day.* Baltimore, Md.: Johns Hopkins University Press (rev. ed.), 1991. The classic self-help book for families and caregivers.

Personal Account

McGowin, Diana. *Living in the Labyrinth: A Personal Journey through the Maze of Alzheimer's.* New York: Dell, 1994. The story of early Alzheimer's disease, told from the perspective of an afflicted individual.

Advocacy Movement

Alzheimer's Association (National Headquarters), 919 North Michigan Avenue, Suite 1000, Chicago, IL 60611-1676; 1-800-272-3900. Publishes a monthly newsletter with information for families and caregivers; local chapters have information on support groups and other community services for individuals with Alzheimer's and their families.

Government Resources

Alzheimer's Disease Education and Referral Center (a service of the National Institute on Aging), P.O. Box 8250, Silver Spring, MD 20907-8250; 1-800-438-4380. Publishes an annual update on the science of Alzheimer's and can supply information about ongoing research at the twenty-eight federally funded Alzheimer's Disease Research Centers.

Fictional Account

Ignatieff, Michael. *Scar Tissue.* New York: Farrar, Straus, and Giroux, 1994. A contemporary novel about Alzheimer's.

Science

Terry, Robert; Katzman, Robert; and Bick, Katherine, eds. *Alzheimer Disease.* New York: Raven Press, 1994. For the technically inclined, a superb compendium of articles on all aspects of the science of Alzheimer's.

History

Pollen, Daniel. *Hannah's Heirs: The Quest for the Genetic Origins of Alzheimer's Disease.* New York: Oxford University Press (revised and expanded), 1996. A good but technical account of the search for Alzheimer genes.

Ethics

Post, Stephen. *The Moral Challenge of Alzheimer's Disease.* Baltimore: Johns Hopkins University Press, 1995. An extended essay on the ethical issues associated with dementia.

Attitudes Toward Aging

Cole, Thomas. *The Journey of Life: A Cultural History of Aging in America.* New York; Cambridge University Press, 1991. A history of attitudes toward aging as reflected primarily in art and literature in America.

Data

Office of Technology Assessment Task Force. *Losing a Million Minds: Confronting the Tragedy of Alzheimer's Disease and Other Dementias.* Philadelphia: J. B. Lippincott, 1987. Many useful statistics relating to dementia.

Notes

■ Introduction

1. Quoted in Jaber Gubrium, *Oldtimers and Alzheimer's: The Descriptive Organization of Senility* (Greenwich, Conn.: Jai Alai Press, 1986).

2. Matthew Spetalnick, "Reagan Discloses He Has Alzheimer's Disease," Reuters, November 5, 1994.

3. Elizabeth Bumiller, "Effects of Reagan Illness Detailed," *Boston Globe*, June 8, 1995, p. 3.

4. Alzheimer's Association news releases: March 13, 1996, and March 27, 1996.

5. Quoted in Jeff Lyon and Peter Gorner, *Altered Fates: Gene Therapy and the Retooling of Human Life* (New York: Norton, 1995), p. 446.

6. Lewis Thomas, *Late Night Thoughts on Listening to Mahler's Ninth Symphony* (New York: Viking, 1983).

7. U.S. Department of Health and Human Services, Public Health Service Agency for Health Care Policy and Research, Rockville, Md. P. Costa, T. Williams, M. Somerfield, et al., "Recognition and Initial Assessment of Alzheimer's Disease and Related Dementias," *Clinical Practice Guideline No. 19*, no. 97-0702 (November 1996). Other authorities claim as many as four million Americans have Alzheimer's disease, which implies more than six million have some form of dementia. Recognizing that estimates are made by investigators, based on their methodology, I prefer to err on the low side and have chosen the conservative estimate used by the Agency for Health Care Policy and Research.

8. A recent book addressing chiefly the economic and legal ramifications of an aging society is Richard Posner, *Aging and Old Age* (Chicago:

University of Chicago Press, 1995). The leading work arguing for an intergenerational perspective is by the philosopher Norman Daniels, *Just Health Care* (New York: Cambridge University Press, 1985). The major—and eloquent—exponent of the view that there is more to life than health and that meaning rather than longevity should be the major goal of new policies toward aging is Daniel Callahan. See *Setting Limits: Medical Goals in an Aging Society* (New York: Simon & Schuster, 1987).

9. Estimates are that the Medicare trust fund will go bankrupt in 2002 if current demands remain unchanged.

10. I take a stab at this more general problem in my previous book, *Choosing Medical Care in Old Age: What Kind, How Much, When to Stop* (Cambridge, Mass.: Harvard University Press, 1994).

11. Elisabeth Kübler-Ross, *On Death and Dying* (New York: Macmillan, 1969).

12. Sherwin Nuland, *How We Die* (New York: Knopf, 1994).

13. See Charles Rosenberg, "Framing Illness, Society, and History," in C. Rosenberg, *Explaining Epidemics and Other Studies in the History of Medicine* (New York: Cambridge University Press, 1991), pp. 305–18. Rosenberg argues that "we need to know more about the individual experience of disease in time and place, the influence of culture on definitions of disease and of disease in the creation of culture, and the role of the state in defining and responding to disease."

■ CHAPTER 1: *Sunset*

1. There are a host of screening tests for dementia, including the Dementia Test Score, the Short Portable Mental Status Questionnaire, and the Folstein Mini-Mental State. The commonly used tests, as well as recommended laboratory tests, are described in A. Siu, "Screening for Dementia and Investigating Its Causes," *Annals of Internal Medicine* 115 (1991): 122–32. The most widely used test, so commonly employed that it is often simply known as *the* mini-mental status exam (MMSE), was first reported in M. Folstein, B. Folstein, and P. McHugh, "Mini-Mental State: A Practical Method for Grading the Cognitive State of Patients for the Clinician," *Journal of Psychiatry Research* 12 (1975): 189–98.

2. A widely quoted study revealing the rarity with which American physicians used to reveal a cancer diagnosis to their patients is D. Oken, "What to Tell the Cancer Patient," *Journal of the American Medical Association* 175 (1961): 1120–8. A follow-up study was reported eighteen years later: D. Novack, R. Plumer, R. Smith, et al., "Changes in Physicians' Attitudes Towards Telling the Cancer Patient," *Journal of the American Medical Association* 241 (1979): 897–900. By this time, most physicians reported full disclosure.

3. An analysis of the problems of truth-telling when the diagnosis is dementia is to be found in M. Drickamer and M. Lachs, "Should Patients with Alzheimer's Disease Be Told Their Diagnosis?" *New England Journal of Medicine* 326 (1992): 947–51.

4. For a discussion of the case of Janet Adkins, the Oregon woman who sought out Jack Kevorkian in response to her dementia, see K. Rohde, E. Peskind, and M. Raskind, "Suicide in Two Patients with Alzheimer's Disease," *Journal of the American Geriatrics Society* 43 (1995): 187–89. For a description of Dr. Kevorkian's approach to assisted suicide and an analysis of why it is neither medical nor ethical, see George Annas, "Physician-Assisted Suicide: Michigan's Temporary Solution," *New England Journal of Medicine* 328 (1993): 1573–76.

5. Clinical criteria for diagnosing Alzheimer's disease were formally established only in 1984, through the joint efforts of an NIH agency and a private agency, the National Institute of Neurological Diseases and Stroke and the Alzheimer's Disease and Related Disorders Association. Their recommendations were published as G. McKhann, D. Drachman, M. Folstein, et al., "Clinical Diagnosis of Alzheimer's Disease: Report of the NINCDS-ADRDA Work Group Under the Auspices of the Department of Health and Human Services Task Force on Alzheimer's Disease," *Neurology* 34 (1984): 1939–49.

6. The subject of elderly drivers, and in particular of elderly drivers with dementia, is well reviewed by L. Hunt in her chapter, "Driving and the Demented Person," in John Morris, ed., *Handbook of Dementing Illnesses* (New York: Marcel Dekker, 1994) pp. 528–38.

■ CHAPTER 2: *Alzheimer's Disease—the Science*

1. In 1995, the *New England Journal of Medicine* had two articles about the science of Alzheimer's disease. The first, in the section entitled Clinical Implications of Basic Research, dealt with a possible animal model for Alzheimer's disease: Rudolph Tanzi, "A Promising Animal Model of Alzheimer's Disease," *New England Journal of Medicine* 332 (1995): 1512–13. The second was an ambitious study in the Original Articles section, which correlated genetic analysis of blood samples, clinical evaluations of patients, and pathologic examination of autopsy specimens in individuals over eight-five years of age: T. Polvikosk, R. Sulkava, M. Haltia, et al., "Apolipoprotein E, Dementia, and Cortical Deposition of Beta-amyloid Protein," *New England Journal of Medicine* 333 (1995): 1242–47.

2. Amyloid was first identified in 1853 by the pathologist Rudolf Virchow. Best known for recognizing the cell as the fundamental unit of health and disease, Virchow was a passionate microscopist. Whenever possible, he sought to relate his observations to the functions of organs. Sometimes

he made discoveries that remained inexplicable for years to come. One such finding was the accumulation of thin threads or filaments outside of cells. When he noticed the same deposits in a variety of organs, in numerous diseases, he decided to call them "amyloid," meaning starch-like. Virchow, with his customary insight, concluded that this mysterious material was, in some unclear way, gumming up the works. Over the years, amyloid was found in a variety of organs in the body and was associated with several distinct disease processes. The Belgian Paul Divry wrote a paper describing the optical properties of amyloid, in 1927. A subsequent paper of his in 1934 reported that amyloid was the stuff in Redlich's plaques and was Alzheimer's "peculiar substance."

3. R. Terry, N. Gonatas, and M. Weiss, "Ultrastructural Studies in Alzheimer's Presenile Dementia," *American Journal of Pathology* 44 (1964): 269–81.

4. Jean Marx, "Alzheimer's Debate Boils Over," *Science* 257 (1992): 1336–68.

5. For an accessible description, see Wade Roush, "Protein Studies Try to Puzzle Out Alzheimer's Tangles," *Science* 267 (1995): 783–84. The work describing the "hyperphosphorylation" of tau is A. Alonso, T. Zaidi, I. Grundke-Iqbal, and K. Iqbal, "Role of Abnormal Phosphory-lated Tau in the Breakdown of Microtubules in Alzheimer's Disease," *Proceedings of the National Academy of Sciences* 91 (1994): 5562–66.

6. See Jean Marx, "Alzheimer's Pathology Explained," *Science* 249 (1990): 984–86 for a description of the work of Kenneth Kosik at Harvard in this area.

7. H. Arai, M. Terajima, M. Miura, et al., "Tau in Cerebrospinal Fluid: A Potential Diagnostic Marker in Alzheimer's Disease," *Annals of Neurology* 38 (1995): 649–52.

8. The story of twilight sleep is told by Judith Leavitt in her history of American childbirth, *Brought to Bed: Child-Bearing in America, 1750–1950* (New York: Oxford University Press, 1986).

9. D. Drachman and L. Leavitt, "Human Memory and the Cholinergic System: A Relationship to Aging?" *Archives of Neurology* 30 (1974): 113–21.

10. The original articles on cholinergic dropout in Alzheimer's are by Davies and Malory and by Bowen et al. A nice summary of the cholinergic theory is by C. Geula and M. Mesulam, "Cholinergic Systems and Related Neuropathological Predilection Patterns in Alzheimer Disease," in Terry, Katzman, Bick, eds., *Alzheimer Disease* (New York: Raven Press, 1994), pp. 263–91.

11. B. Cohen, P. Renshaw, A. Strell, et al., "Decreased Brain Choline Uptake in Older Adults: An In Vivo Proton Magnetic Resonance Spec-

troscopy Study," *Journal of the American Medical Association* 274 (1995): 902–7.

12. For a recent study that details both benefits and risks, see M. Knapp, D. Knopman, P. Solomon, et al., "A 30-Week Randomized Controlled Trial of High-Dose Tacrine in Patients with Alzheimer's Disease," *Journal of the American Medical Association* 271 (1994): 985–91.

13. For an excellent account of the search for the genetic form of Alzheimer's disease, see Daniel Pollen, *Hannah's Heirs: An Account of the Search for the Genetic Basis of Alzheimer's Disease* (New York: Oxford University Press, 1993).

14. The earliest report was by P. St. George-Hyslop, R. Tanzi, R. Polinsky, et al., "The Genetic Defect Causing Familial Alzheimer's Disease Maps on Chromosome 21," *Science* 235 (1987): 885–90.

15. In late 1987 and early 1988, two reports were published of families in which the Alzheimer gene was *not* linked to chromosome 21. One was G. Schellenberg, T. Bird, E. Wijsman, et al., "Absence of Linkage of Chromosome 21q21 Markers to Familial Alzheimer's Disease," *Science* 242 (1988): 1507–10.

16. This race was won by John Hardy and his group, then at St. Mary's Hospital in London. (Hardy subsequently moved to Florida.) A. Goate, M. Charter-Harkin, A. Mullan, et al., "Segregation of Missense Mutation in the Amyloid Precursor Protein Gene with Familial Alzheimer's Disease," *Nature* 349 (1991): 704–6. Only six families worldwide proved to have this particular mutation.

17. Within a six-week period, the same linkage was found by St. George-Hyslop's group in Toronto, by Gerard Schellenberg at the University of Washington, and by Christine Van Broeckhoven in Antwerp, Belgium.

18. The winners of this race were the group under St. George-Hyslop: R. Sherrington, E. Rogaev, Y. Liang, et al., "Cloning of a Gene Bearing Missense Mutation in Early-Onset Familial Alzheimer's Disease," *Nature* 375 (1995): 754–60. There were a total of thirty-three authors listed on this paper.

19. The gene on chromosome 1 was identified by two groups in a one-month period. Priority of publication went to E. Levy-Lahad, E. Wijsnan, E. Nemens, et al., "A Familial Alzheimer's Disease Locus on Chromosome 1," *Science* 269 (1995): 97–103.

20. Marcia Barinaga, "New Alzheimer's Gene Found," *Science* 268 (1995): 1845–46.

21. AP News Service, "Scientists Find Alzheimer Gene," June 28, 1995.

22. The magnitude of the effect is variable. Smoking more than doubles the incidence of coronary disease. Cholesterol risk varies with the

level of cholesterol, but a 10 percent increase in a baseline low-normal risk has been associated with a 21 percent increase in the risk of death. Lowering blood pressure by 5–6 millimeters of mercury has been found to lower the rate of heart attacks by 17 percent. Put another way, each millimeter decrement in blood pressure has been associated with a 2 to 3 percent decrease in risk of death from heart disease. The role of modification of each individual risk factor is discussed in J. Manson, H. Tosteson, P. Ridker, et al., "The Primary Prevention of Myocardial Infarction" (*New England Journal of Medicine* 1992; 326: 1406–16).

23. The role of lifestyle changes in effecting a decline is mortality from heart rate was discussed by L. Goldman and E. Cook in "The Decline in Ischemic Heart Disease Mortality Rates. An Analysis of the Comparative Effects of Medical Interventions and Changes in Lifestyle," *Annals of Internal Medicine* 101 (1984): 825–36. These authors commented on the drop in the death rate from heart disease, which became apparent between 1968 and 1976 (and which has continued since then—falling from a death rate in men of 240/100,000 in 1968 to 110/100,000 in 1988). They estimated that 54 percent of the decline was due to lifestyle changes, as opposed to medical treatment. When they added the contribution of control of blood pressure, a medical treatment but one that addresses a risk factor, they found another 8.5 percent of the decline was due to modifiable factors.

24. John Travis, "New Piece in Alzheimer's Puzzle," *Science* 261 (1993): 828–29.

25. Quoted in Paul Cotton, "Constellation of Risks and Processes Seen in Search for Alzheimer's Clues," *Journal of the American Medical Association* 27 (1994): 89–91.

26. S. Seshadri, D. Drachman, and C. Lippy, "Apoprotein E-ε4 Allele and the Lifetime Risk of Alzheimer's Disease," *Archives of Neurology* 52 (1995): 1074–79.

27. The same issues arise with predictive tests for any of the late-onset neurodegenerative diseases. See T. Bird and R. Bennett, "Why Do DNA Testing? Practical and Ethical Implications of New Neurogenetic Tests," *Annals of Neurology* 38 (1995): 141–46.

28. The article is "Statement on Use of Apolipoprotein E Testing for Alzheimer's Disease," *Journal of the American Medical Association* 274 (1995): 1627–29. The organizations endorsing the statement were: the American Society of Human Genetics, the American Academy of Neurology, the American Psychiatric Association, and the National Institutes of Health—Department of Education Working Group on Ethical, Legal, and Social Implications of Human Genome Research.

29. Thomas Kuhn, *The Structure of Scientific Revolutions* (Chicago: University of Chicago Press, 2nd ed.), 1970.

30. The various aspects of the aluminum story are told by W. Markesbery and W. Ehemann in "Brain Trace Elements and Alzheimer Disease," in R. Terry, R. Katzman, and K. Bick, eds., *Alzheimer Disease* (New York: Raven Press, 1994), pp. 353–67.

31. One of the early articles linking anti-inflammatory medications used in arthritis and a low prevalence of Alzheimer's was M. L. Jenkinson, M. R. Bliss, A. T. Brain, and D. L. Scott, "Rheumatoid Arthritis and Senile Dementia of the Alzheimer Type," *British Journal of Rheumatology* 28 (1988): 86-88.

32. J. Rogers, L. Kirby, S. Hempelman, et al., "Clinical Trial of Indomethacin in Alzheimer's Disease," *Neurology* 43 (1993): 1609-11. Most other studies of anti-inflammatory medication and Alzheimer's do not examine the utility of the drugs for treatment; rather they look at whether this medication, when given for some other reason, seems to lead to a lower rate of Alzheimer's disease. This one study was a randomized trial that found a lower rate of cognitive decline in those on the medication than in those on placebo.

33. The American study looking at this question is A. Paganini-Hill and V. Henderson, "Estrogen Replacement Therapy and Risk of Alzheimer's Disease," *Archives of Internal Medicine* 156 (1996): 2213–17.

34. The report is M. Sano, C. Ernesto, R. Thomas, et al. for the Members of the Alzheimer's Disease Collaborative Study, "A Controlled Trial of Selegeline, Alpha-Tocopherol, or Both as Treatment for Alzheimer's Disease," *New England Journal of Medicine* 336 (1997): 1216–22. Numerous objections to the study have been raised, including the observation that the promising conclusions do not hold up except when certain statisical adjustments are made in the data. In addition, the way of defining the success of a drug was unusual: the two drugs were compared to each other and to placebo in terms of their ability to prolong the time to death *or* nursing home placement *or* development of severe dementia *or* loss of the ability to perform two out of three particular activities of daily living.

35. See D. Snowdon, L. Greiner, J. Mortimer, et al., "Brain Infarction and the Clinical Expression of Alzheimer Disease," *Journal of the American Medical Association* 277 (1977): 813–17. This was one of the growing number of tantalizing findings from what is often called "the nun study," in which members of the School Sisters of Notre Dame agreed to neuropsychological testing during life and autopsies at the time of death. By the end of 1995, 161 of the participating nuns had died. Complete data were available on 102, of whom 61 met the pathologic criteria for Alzheimer's disease. While women with strokes and plaques and tangles had poorer cognitive function than women with plaques and tangles but no strokes, strokes alone were only weakly

associated with dementia in those nuns who did not meet the criteria for Alzheimer's.

36. Extensive clusters of the new lesions were found in the brains of forty people who had had Alzheimer's and very little was found in forty-one people with other forms of dementia. The news media reported widely on the discovery. See Rebecca Voelker, "Quick Uptakes: New Alzheimer Clue," *Journal of the American Medical Association* 278 (1997): 275. This report cites researchers at the National Institute on Aging as saying, "They are hopeful the finding will spur new research and perhaps new treatments."

37. Jean Marx, "Nerve Growth Factor and Alzheimer's: Hopes and Fears," *Science* 247 (1991): 408–10.

38. Marcia Barinaga, "Neurotrophic Factors Enter the Clinic," *Science* 264 (1994): 772–74.

39. In fact, the adequacy of reductionism is being called into question, even for infectious diseases: as tuberculosis rates rise again, it is apparent that antibiotics alone are not enough to eradicate TB. Their efficacy is limited by the capacity of bacteria to develop resistance and by the ability of the person's immune system to work with antibiotics to fend off infection. The virus causing AIDS was identified in 1984, and we are still quite a way from the eradication of that disease.

■ CHAPTER 3: *Twilight*

1. A good summary of the behavioral symptoms of Alzheimer's disease is in the chapter by Marshal Folstein and Frederick Bylsma entitled "Noncognitive Symptoms of Alzheimer Disease," in R. Terry, R. Katzman, and K. Bick, *Alzheimer Disease* (New York: Raven Press, 1994), pp. 27–40. They point out that delusions—false ideas that are "impervious to persuasion, are idiosyncratic and preoccupying, and affect the person's behavior"—occur in 40 percent of Alzheimer patients at some point during their illness. The delusion that someone is stealing from them occurs most commonly; another delusional process involves misidentification—mistaking one person for another. The study looking at the frequency of delusions is L. Deutsch, F. Bylsma, B. Rovner, et al., "Psychosis and Physical Aggression in Probable Alzheimer's Disease," *American Journal of Psychiatry* 148 (1991): 1159–63.

2. See L. Schneider, V. Pollock, and S. Lyness, "A Meta-analysis of Controlled Trials of Neuroleptic Treatment in Dementia," *Journal of the American Geriatrics Society* 38 (1990): 353–63. These authors found only seven double-blind, randomized trials comparing neuroleptics to placebo in patients with agitated dementia. In most of the studies, between one third and one half of patients did improve when treated

with antipsychotic medication, though many also improved with a placebo (sugar pills).

3. See M. Beers, J. Avorn, S. Soumerai, and D. Everitt, "Psychoactive Medication Use in Intermediate Care Facility Residents," *Journal of the American Medical Association* (1988): 3016–20.

4. The percentage of hip fracture patients discharged to nursing homes rose from 38 to 60 after the institution of the DRG system. The percentage of patients remaining in the nursing home one year later rose from 9 to 33 percent. See J. Fitzgerald, P. Moore, and R. Dittus, "The Care of Elderly Patients with Hip Fracture: Changes Since Implementation of the Prospective Payment System," *New England Journal of Medicine* 319 (1988): 1392–97.

5. Memory is a very complex phenomenon. Not so long ago, scientists believed that memory is something frozen into our brains, perhaps first stored in a compartment called short-term memory and then transferred to a permanent storage vault called long-term memory. Remembering, in this model, simply involves retrieval and the only way to lose memories is for the memory banks to be destroyed or damaged. In fact, the truth is much more complicated. The "engram" that is encoded in the brain includes emotions associated with an experience, as well as images and perhaps our impressions of the initial event. Though distinct parts of the brain play unique roles in memory (the hippocampus is involved with encoding new events, and the frontal lobes with retrieval), the entire process depends on networks of neurons that connect the various components. An excellent description of the contemporary understanding of memory and of the experiments that underlie our knowledge is Daniel Schacter's *Searching for Memory: The Brain, the Mind, and the Past* (New York: Basic Books, 1996).

6. The neurologic term for this is "executive function." Impairments in executive function often explain why families suspect something is amiss even when their relative performs quite well on such simple tests of cognitive function as the mini-mental status examination.

■ CHAPTER 4: *Alzheimer's Disease—the History*

1. Quoted in George Rosen, *Madness in Society* (New York: Harper and Row, 1968).

2. Stanley Finger, *Origins of Neuroscience: A History of Explorations into Brain Function* (New York: Oxford University Press, 1994).

3. From Cicero's *De Senectute*, as quoted by Roy Porter, "Dementia," in George Berrios and Roy Porter, eds., *A History of Clinical Psychiatry: The Origin and History of Psychiatric Disorders* (New York: New York University Press), 1995, pp. 52–64.

4. Ibid.

5. William Shakespeare, *As You Like It,* II: vii.

6. See Charles Rosenberg, "Body and Mind in Nineteenth-Century Medicine: Some Clinical Origins of the Neurosis Construct," in Charles Rosenberg, *Explaining Epidemics* (New York: Cambridge University Press, 1978), pp. 74–89.

7. An important essay that examines the development of the idea of specificity of disease is by Charles Rosenberg, "Disease and Social Order in America: Perceptions and Expectations," in Charles Rosenberg, *Explaining Epidemics* (New York: Cambridge University Press, 1992), pp. 258–77.

8. Richard Torack, "The Early History of Senile Dementia," in Barry Reisberg, ed., *Alzheimer's Disease* (New York: The Free Press, 1983), pp. 23–27.

9. A good discussion of Pinel's contribution is to be found in Gerald Grob, *The Mad Among Us: A History of the Care of American Mentally Ill* (New York: The Free Press, 1994).

10. Jean Esquirol, *Mental Maladies: Treatise on Insanity.* Translated with additions by E. K. Hunt, M.D. (Philadelphia: Lea and Blanchard, 1845). The original French edition was published in 1838.

11. Alois Alzheimer, "On a Peculiar Disease of the Cerebral Cortex," a translation of "Uber eine Eigenartige Erkrankung der Hirnrinde." *Allgemeine Zeitschrift für Psychiatrie und Psychisch-Gerichtlich Medizin* 64 (1911): 146–48, printed in Neurological Classics XX, *Archives of Neurology* 21 (1969): 809–10.

12. Alois Alzheimer, "On Certain Peculiar Diseases of Old Age," a translation of "Uber Eigenartige Krankheitsfalle des Spaeteren Alters." *Zeitschrift für die gesamte Neurologie und Psychiatrie* 4 (1911): 4: 356–85, printed in the journal *History of Psychiatry* 2 (1991): 74–99.

13. Emil Kraepelin, *Psychiatrie. Ein Lehrbuch fuer Studierende und Aertze. II. Band. Klinische Psychiatrie* (Leipzig: Verlag von Johann Ambrosius Barth, 1910).

14. Kraepelin's *Lectures on Clinical Psychiatry* (Revised and edited by Thomas Johnstone; facsimile of 1904 edition published by Hafner Publication Company, New York, 1968).

15. Emil Kraepelin, *Psychiatrie. Ein Lehrbuch fuer Studierende und Aertze. II. Band. Klinische Psychiatrie* (Leipzig: Verlag von Johann Ambrosius Barth, 1910).

16. The original case discussion was presented to the American and Canadian Medical Associations on June 12, 1935; it was published in

the *Canadian Medical Association Journal* in 1936, 35: 361–66, and reprinted in an article by J. Hanna, "A Case of Alzheimer's Disease with Neuropathological Findings" in the *Canadian Medical Association Journal* 145 (1991): 823–29.

17. One possible explanation for the decision to regard Alzheimer's disease as a disease of middle age is the rivalry between two schools of pathology: that in Munich (where Alzheimer worked at the Psychiatric and Neurologic Clinic directed by Kraepelin), and that in Prague (where Emil Fischer worked at the German Psychiatric Clinic, directed by Pick). Alzheimer discovered tangles, and Fischer and Redlich described plaques. Alzheimer found tangles in the brain of a fifty-four-year-old woman with clinical dementia and concluded the tangles were a quintessential pathologic feature of the disease. Fisher found plaques in twelve out of sixteen cases of senile dementia (but in no cases of syphilitic controls) and concluded that plaques were specific for dementia. According to the competing schools theory, if Alzheimer had announced that his tangles were merely another microscopic abnormality of senile dementia, his discovery would have met with little interest. Only by treating the tangles as the basis of a totally new disease would the discovery have been deemed important. I am not convinced that finding a second feature of a disease would have been ignored. Moreover, this theory implies that the early twentieth century gave birth to two new diseases: Alzheimer's disease (a dementing illness in those under sixty) and Fischer's disease (a dementing illness in those over sixty). In fact, no Fischer's disease was recognized. Far more plausible is that neuropathologists *assumed* that cognitive decline in the elderly was part of normal aging. They were so convinced that memory loss, wandering, and language difficulties demanded an explanation when they arose in a fifty-year-old but not when they developed in a seventy-year-old that they distorted their own observations to fit the categories they believed existed. See Luigi Amaducci, Walter Rocca, and Bruce Schoenberg, "Origins of the Distinction Between Alzheimer's Disease and Senile Dementia: How History Can Clarify Nosology," *Neurology* 36 (1986): 1497–99.

18. Quoted in Carole Haber, *Beyond Sixty-Five* (New York: Cambridge University Press, 1983), p. 75.

19. George Beard, *American Nervousness: Its Causes and Consequences* (New York: Putnam, 1881).

20. See I. L. Nascher, *Geriatrics: The Diseases of Old Age and Their Treatment* (Philadelphia: Blakiston's Sons and Co., 1914).

21. Another very persuasive factor was Kraepelin's decision to come down in favor of the two-disease model. Kraepelin was a very highly respect nosologist. See Martha Holstein, "Alzheimer's Disease and Senile Dementia, 1885–1920: An Interpretive History of Disease Negotiation," *Journal of Aging Studies*, in press.

22. I. L. Nascher, *Geriatrics: The Diseases of Old Age and Their Treatment* (Philadelphia: Blakiston's Sons and Co., 1914).

23. Walford Thewlis, *Geriatrics: A Treatise on Senile Conditions, Diseases of Advanced Life, and Care of the Aged* (St. Louis, Missouri: Mosby, 1919).

24. Argued in Thomas Cole, *The Journey of Life: A Cultural History of Aging in America* (New York: Cambridge University Press, 1992).

25. In this and much of what follows, I am indebted to Thomas Cole.

26. The reference is to Titus 2:20.

27. David Fischer, *Growing Old in America* (New York: Oxford University Press, 1978).

28. Andrew Achenbaum, *Old Age in the New Land* (Baltimore, Md.: Johns Hopkins University Press, 1978). Achenbaum and Fischer offer differing interpretations of when old age acquired a bad name in America. Achenbaum puts the break after the Civil War; Fischer argues it came around the turn of the century.

29. For a delightful account of the nineteenth-century health reformers, see James Whorton, *Crusaders for Fitness: A History of American Health Reformers* (Princeton, N.J.: Princeton University Press, 1982).

30. Thomas Cole, *The Journey of Life: A Cultural History of Aging in America* (New York: Cambridge University Press, 1992).

31. George Day, *A Practical Treatise on the Domestic Management and Most Important Diseases of Advanced Life* (Philadelphia: Lea and Blanchard, 1849).

32. Elmer Lee, "The Frequency of Apoplexy Among the Higher Classes with Suggestions for Its Prevention and Escape from Fatality," *Journal of the American Medical Association* 30 (1898): 1083–84.

33. W. Hammond, *A Treatise on the Diseases of the Nervous System* (New York: Appleton and Company, 1892).

34. George Beard, *American Nervousness: Its Causes and Consequences* (New York: Putnam, 1881), p. 194.

35. See Daniel Boorstin, *The Americans: The Democratic Experience* (New York: Random House, 1973), for a description of go-getters in nineteenth-century American society.

36. Charles Stephens, *Natural Salvation* (Norway Lake: Maine, 1903).

37. Henry Thoreau, *Walden* (New York: Anchor Press/Doubleday, 1973), p. 12.

38. Such a selective sampling of nineteenth century literature can obviously be misleading. However, a thorough review by David Fischer,

op cit, who quotes the line from Whitman, finds these examples to be representative.

39. Two landmark studies in the psychiatric literature daringly concluded that the emperor wore no clothes—that presenile dementia and senile dementia were indistinguishable. The first was by R. Newton, "The Identity of Alzheimer's Disease and Senile Dementia and Their Relationship to Senility," *British Journal of Psychiatry* (1948) 94: 225–49. The second, appearing in an American journal, was M. Neumann and R. Cohn, "Incidence of Alzheimer's Disease in a Large Mental Hospital: Relation to Senile Psychosis and Psychosis with Cerebral Arteriosclerosis," *Archives of Neurology and Psychiatry* (1953) 69: 615–36.

40. J. Tanur, F. Mosteller, W. Kruskal, et al., eds., *Statistics: A Guide to the Unknown* (San Francisco: Holden-Day, 1978).

41. The British triumvirate published their work in two critical articles: G. Blessed, B. Tomlinson, and M. Roth, "The Association Between Quantitative Measures of Dementia and of Senile Changes in the Cerebral Grey Matter of Elderly Subjects," *British Journal of Psychiatry* (1968) 114: 792–811, and, two years later: B. Tomlinson, G. Blessed, and M. Roth, "Observations on the Brains of Demented Old People," *Journal of Neurological Science* (1970) 11: 205–42.

42. Peter Laslett, "Necessary Knowledge: Age and Ageing in the Societies of the Past," in D. Kertzer and P. Laslett, eds., *Aging in the Past: Demography, Society, and Old Age* (Berkeley: University of California Press, 1995), pp. 3–77.

43. Laslett suggests that a society has entered the Third Age when at least half its population can be expected to survive from age twenty-five to age seventy and when at least a quarter of all adults, defined as twenty-five and over, are beyond the age of sixty. See Laslett, op. cit.

44. Joint National Committee, "The 1988 Report of the Joint National Committee on Detection, Evaluation, and Treatment of High Blood Pressure," *Archives of Internal Medicine* 148 (1988): 1023–48.

45. The observation that elderly people do not typically *feel* old, or indeed any different from how they felt at a younger age, is brought home by Sharon Kaufman in *The Ageless Self: Sources of Meaning in Late Life* (Madison: University of Wisconsin Press, 1986).

■ CHAPTER 5: *Evening Star*

1. Reminiscence therapy is controversial but its proponents believe it helps older people find meaning in a society that tends to devalue them. See Florence Soltys and Larue Coats, "The SolCos Model: Facilitating Reminiscence Therapy," *Journal of Gerontological Nursing* 20 (1994): 11–16.

2. A discussion of the history of the care of the elderly, and an argument for the benefits of institutional care, as opposed to community care, is to be found in Muriel R. Gillick, "Long-Term Care Options for the Frail Elderly," *Journal of the American Geriatrics Society* 37 (1989): 1198–1203.

3. Tacrine first hit the medical literature in the form of an article in a prestigious journal reporting the results of a very small study done by little-known investigators. (W. Summers, L. Majorski, G. Marsh, et al., "Oral Tetrahydroaminoacridine in Long-Term Treatment of Senile Dementia, Alzheimer Type," *New England Journal of Medicine* 315 [1986]: 1241–45.) This preliminary report led to the establishment of a multicenter study of tacrine. The first report of the group failed to show any beneficial effect of tacrine (K. Davis, L. Thal, E. Gamzu, et al., "A Double-Blind, Placebo-Controlled Multicenter Study of Tacrine for Alzheimer's Disease," *New England Journal of Medicine* 327 [1992]: 1253–59). However, this study was criticized for failing to use sufficiently high doses. A subsequent study did present persuasive evidence for the existence of slight benefit in those individuals who could tolerate high doses (M. Farlow, S. Graem, L. Hershey, et al., "A Controlled Trial of Tacrine in Alzheimer's Disease," *Journal of the American Medical Association* 268 [1992]: 2523–29).

4. The study is in D. Knopman, L. Schneider, K. Davis, et al., "Long-term Tacrine (Cognex) Treatment: Effects on Nursing Home Placement and Mortality," *Neurology* 47 (1996): 166–77. After patients completed the randomized double-blind placebo phase of the Tacrine Study Group trial, they were allowed to continue on tacrine. Six hundred and sixty such patients were followed for at least two years. Those who remained on tacrine and received doses of greater than eighty milligrams a day were less likely to enter a nursing home.

5. M. Sano, C. Ernesto, R. Thomas, et al., for the Members of the Alzheimer's Disease Collaborative Study, "A Controlled Trial of Selegeline, Alpha-Tocopherol, or Both as Treatment for Alzheimer's Disease," *New England Journal of Medicine* 336 (1997): 1216–22. Alpha-Tocopherol is vitamin E. For a discussion of the shortcomings of this study, see Chapter 2 on the science of Alzheimer's disease.

6. A recent discussion of the ethics of doing research in individuals with dementia is to be found in G. Sachs, C. Stocking, R. Stein, et al., "Ethical Aspects of Dementia Research. Informed Consent and Proxy Consent," *Clinical Research* 42 (1994): 403–12.

■ **CHAPTER 6:** *Alzheimer's Disease—the Politics*

1. Robert Katzman, "The Prevalence and Malignancy of Alzheimer Disease, a Major Killer," *Archives of Neurology* 33 (1976): 217–18.

2. Paul Starr, *The Social Transformation of American Medicine* (New York: Basic Books, 1982)

3. From the Civil War to World War I, full-time academic research and teaching positions were rare in the United States. Young American physicians interested in research had to travel abroad, typically to Germany, to train, and on their return sometimes found they could not pursue research careers unless they were independently wealthy. Between the world wars, medical research established a firm footing in American medical colleges, but it took off after World War II. See Kenneth Ludmerer, *Learning to Heal: The Development of American Medical Education* (New York: Basic Books), 1985.

4. Eli Friedman, "End-Stage Renal Disease Therapy: An American Success Story," *Journal of the American Medical Association* 275 (1996): 1118–22. Not everyone believes the program is a success story. An article in the same issue of *JAMA* suggests that Americans spend far more than other countries on end-stage renal disease, and that they spend far too much (Richard Rettig, "The Social Contract and the Treatment of Permanent Kidney Failure," *Journal of the American Medical Association* 275 [1996]: 1123–26). Parenthetically, the cost of making dialysis available to all Americans with renal failure soared in the first ten years of the program from $229 million to $2 billion. Total costs for the end-stage renal disease program (including both dialysis and kidney transplants) reached $9.5 billion in 1992 (about 5 percent of the total Medicare budget).

5. The debate between the science of aging and the science of the diseases of old age rages on. This is the theme of the book *How and Why We Age* by the noted biologist Leonard Hayflick (New York: Ballantine Books, 1994).

6. Neal Cutler, "Public Response: The National Politics of Alzheimer's Disease," in M. Gilhooly, S. Zarit, and J. Birren, eds., *The Dementias: Policy and Management* (Englewood Cliffs, N.J.: Prentice-Hall, 1986), pp. 161–89, provides the 25,000 figure. In another important article on the politics of Alzheimer's disease, Patrick Fox, "From Senility to Alzheimer's Disease: the Rise of the Alzheimer's Disease Movement," *The Milbank Quarterly* 67 (1989): 58–102 cites a figure of 30,000–40,000. Clearly there was an outpouring of interest.

7. G. McKhann, D. Drachman, M. Folstein, et al., "Clinical Diagnosis of Alzheimer's Disease," Report of the NINCDS-ADRDA Work Group Under the Auspices of the Department of Health and Human Services Task Force on Alzheimer's Disease, *Neurology* (1984) 34: 939–44.

8. W. Andrew Achenbaum, *Crossing Frontiers: Gerontology Emerges as a Science* (New York: Cambridge University Press, 1995). The total NIA budget in 1993 was $401 million.

9. For a detailed description of the development of the Human Genome Project, as well as of the NIH budget process, see Robert Cook-Deegan, *The Gene Wars* (New York: Norton, 1994).

10. Twenty families have been identified with an abnormal gene coding for amyloid precursor protein (located on chromosome 21); three big families have been found with a mutation of the PS2 gene on chromosome 1, and about one hundred families have been found with a mutation of the PS1 gene on chromosome 14. See Writing Committee, Lance Conference, "The Challenge of the Dementias," *Lancet* 347 (1996): 1303–7.

11. James Watson, "A Personal View of the Project," in Daniel Kevles and Leroy Hood, eds., *The Code of Codes* (Cambridge, Mass.: Harvard University Press, 1992), p. 166.

12. The May 19, 1996, issue of the *New York Times Magazine* contained an article by economist Lester Thurow, "Birth of a Revolutionary Class." He argued that entitlement programs, in particular Medicare, will bankrupt the U.S. Of note, the *Times* reported it received about five-hundred letters in response to Thurow's remarks.

13. A good history of disease politics is Stephen Strickland, *Politics, Science, and Dread Disease: A Short History of United States Medical Research Policy* (Cambridge, Mass.: Harvard University Press, 1972).

14. Gene Cohen, "Alzheimer's Disease: Current Policy Initiatives," in Binstock, Post, and Whitehouse, eds., *Dementia and Aging* (Baltimore, Md., Johns Hopkins University Press, 1992), pp. 171–80.

15. Several commentators believe that the medicalization of deviance—explaining and treating personal and social problems as medical problems—has many unfortunate consequences: once an individual is labeled as having Alzheimer's, there may be a self-fulfilling prophecy of impairment; behavioral problems of the individual with cognitive decline are attributed to the disease instead of to "problems in the caregiver relationship." See Ann Robertson, "The Politics of Alzheimer's Disease: A Case Study in Apocalyptic Demography," *International Journal of Health Services* 20 (1994): 429–42; Karen Lyman, "On the Biomedicalization of Dementia," *The Gerontologist* 29 (1989): 597–605; and Jaber Gubrium, *Oldtimers and Alzheimer's: The Descriptive Organization of Senility* (Greenwich, Conn.: Jai Alai Press, 1986).

16. Quoted in Teri Randall, "Is it 'Oldtimer's Disease' or Just Growing Old?" *Journal of the American Medical Association* 265 (1991): 310–11.

17. Writing Committee, Lancet Conference, "The Challenge of the Dementias," *Lancet* 347 (1996): 1303–7.

18. P. Harrison, "S 182: From Worm Sperm to Alzheimer's Disease," *Lancet* 346 (1995): 388.

19. Richard Adelman, "The Alzheimerization of Aging," *The Gerontologist* 35 (1995): 526–32.

20. W. Summers, L. Majovski, G. Marsh, et al., "Oral Tetrahydroaminoacridine in Long-Term Treatment of Senile Dementia, Alzheimer's Type," *New England Journal of Medicine* 315 (1986): 1241–45.

21. Kenneth Davis and Richard Mohs, "Cholinergic Drugs in Alzheimer's Disease," *New England Journal of Medicine* 315 (1986) 1286–87.

22. William Summers et al., "Use of THA in treatment of Alzheimer-Like Dementia: Pilot Study in Twelve Patients," *Biological Psychiatry* 16 (1981): 145–53.

23. Food and Drug Administration, "An Interim Report from the FDA," *New England Journal of Medicine* 324 (1991): 349–52.

24. Robert Wachter, "AIDS, Activism, and the Politics of Health," *New England Journal of Medicine* 326 (1992): 128–33.

25. K. Davis, L. Thal, E. Gamzu, et al., "A Double-Blind, Placebo-Controlled Multicenter Study of Tacrine for Alzheimer's Disease," *New England Journal of Medicine* 327 (1992): 1253–59.

26. John Growdon, "Treatment for Alzheimer's Disease?" *New England Journal of Medicine* 327 (1992): 1306–8.

27. M. Knapp, D. Knopman, P. Solomon, et al., for the Tacrine Study Group, "A 30-Week Randomized Controlled Trial of High-Dose Tacrine in Patients with Alzheimer's Disease," *Journal of the American Medical Association* 271 (1994): 985–91. Actually, the story is even more complicated. In 1992, yet another tacrine study was published, also by the Tacrine Study Group. Their results emanated from 23 medical centers and 468 patients. These authors also used many scales to measure cognitive function, in addition to an overall assessment of performance. In patients receiving the higher of the two doses tried, 51 percent demonstrated improvement. (M. Farlow, S. Gracon, L. Hershey, et al. for the Tacrine Study Group, "A Controlled Trial of Tacrine in Alzheimer's Disease," *Journal of the American Medical Association* 268 [1992]: 2523–29.) Based on the results of this earlier study, the FDA had announced that tacrine was approved as an investigational drug to be used in treatment protocols. This is a strategy invoked by the FDA to allow patients with very serious diseases for which there is no available treatment to obtain a new drug before it meets criteria for market approval, provided their physicians adhere to certain specified criteria. (See Stuart Nightingale, " From the Food and Drug Administration," *Journal of the American Medical Association* 267 [1992]: 339.) Full approval of the drug came when the second Tacrine Study Group results became available.

28. Cited by Daniel Kevles and Leroy Hood in their reflections on the Human Genome Project in Kevles and Hood, eds., *The Code of Codes* (Cambridge, Mass.: Harvard University Press, 1992). They also comment that much of the literature on DNA sequencing is in the form of patents, not journal articles.

29. C. Joachim, H. Mori, and D. Selkoe, "Amyloid Beta-Protein Deposition in Tissue Other Than Brain in Alzheimer's Disease," *Nature* 341 (1989): 226–30.

30. L. Scinto, K. Daffner, D. Dressler, et al., "Potential Noninvasive Neurobiological Test for Alzheimer's Disease," *Science* 266 (1994): 1051–54.

31. The results of the unpublished studies, studies which have therefore not been subjected to peer review, are included in the company literature. See Joan Stephenson, "Alzheimer Disease Experts Advise a 'Wait for the Data' Response to New Diagnostic Test," *Journal of the American Medical Association* 227 (1997): 870.

32. The desirability of identifying who is at very high risk of breast cancer is controversial. Since there is no effective means of *prevention* and there is a considerable risk of developing the disease even among women who *do not* have the BRCA1 or BRCA2 genes (the genes associated with breast and ovarian cancers), many thoughtful physicians and ethicists are opposed to screening for breast cancer.

33. Medical journals require that authors disclose possible conflicts of interest. Roses in his work on *APOE* has indicated that he has a patent application pending for use of *APOE* genotyping in the diagnosis and prediction of Alzheimer's. Athena Neurosciences holds an option on licensing this patent. Athena Neurosciences bought Genica, a laboratory offering *APOE* testing and reporting protocols to aid physicians in the diagnosis of dementia. Roses has a financial interest in Athena. See the disclosure following Allen Roses's article, "Apoprotein E Genotyping in the Differential Diagnosis, Not Prediction, of Alzheimer's Disease," *Annals of Neurology* 38 (1995): 6–14.

34. The discovery was reported on by Jean Marx, "New 'Alzheimer's Mouse' Produced," *Science* 274 (1996): 172–78. The original article is by K. Hsiao, P. Chapman, S. Nilsen, et al., "Correlative Memory Deficits, Aβ Elevation, and Amyloid Plaques in Transgenic Mice." *Science* 274 (1996): 99–102, from the Department of Neurology at the University of Minnesota.

35. Robert Cook-Deegan, *The Gene Wars* (New York: Norton, 1994).

36. The ethical arguments are spelled out by Henry Greely, "Conflicts in the Biotechnology Industry," *Journal of Law, Medicine, and Ethics* 23 (1995): 354–59.

37. Cited in Robert Cook-Deegan, *The Gene Wars* (New York: Norton, 1994).

38. These shenanigans are reported in the revised and expanded version of Daniel Pollen's book *Hannah's Heirs: The Quest for the Genetic Origins of Alzheimer's Disease* (New York: Oxford University Press, 1996).

39. The entire story is related by Leslie Roberts, "Genome Patent Fight Erupts," *Science* 254 (1991): 184–86.

40. Bernardine Healy, "On Gene Patenting," *New England Journal of Medicine* 327 (1992): 664–68.

41. Rebecca Eisenberg, "Genes, Patents, and Product Development," *Science* 257 (1992): 903–8.

42. The story is told by Cook-Deegan, *The Gene Wars* (New York: Norton, 1994).

43. Thomas Kiley, "Patents on Random Complementary DNA Fragments," *Science* 257 (1992): 915–18.

■ CHAPTER 7: *Nightfall*

1. Incontinence in Alzheimer's disease increases with the severity of the illness. Among mildly affected individuals, the prevalence has been reported to be 5 percent, among moderately affected, 16 percent, and among severely affected, 71 percent. L. Teri, E. Larson, and B. Reifler, "Behavioral Disturbances in Dementia of the Alzheimer's Type," *Journal of the American Geriatrics Society* 36 (1988): 1–6. Other studies have indicated that within six years of diagnosis, 50 percent of individuals will have incontinence and within eight years of diagnosis, 80 percent (Cited in M. Folstein and F. Bylsma, "Noncognitive Symptoms of Alzheimer Disease," in R. Terry, R. Katzman, K. Bick, eds., *Alzheimer Disease* [New York: Raven Press, 1994] pp. 27–40).

2. Neil Resnick, "Urinary Incontinence," *Lancet* 346 (1995): 94–99 provides a good medical summary of the diagnosis and treatment of incontinence.

3. The estrogen story is complicated. Indirect, epidemiologic evidence suggests that postmenopausal women taking estrogen replacement are less likely than women not on estrogen to develop Alzheimer's, and if they do become demented, it is at a later age. Estrogen's benefits, if confirmed in randomized trials that are now in progress, are thought to be due to improvements in blood flow and a protective effect on neurons. The literature is summarized by Ingrid Wickelgren in "Estrogen Stakes Claim to Cognition," *Science* 276 (1997): 675–78.

4. The study was M. Mittelman, S. Ferris, E. Shulman, et al., "A Family Intervention to Delay Nursing Home Placement of Patients with

Alzheimer Disease: A Randomized Controlled Trial," *Journal of the American Medical Association* 276 (1996): 1725–31. The intervention that families received consisted of six sessions of individual and family counseling plus joining a support group. The patients whose families were randomized to the intervention group stayed at home an average of 329 days longer than the controls. Adjustments were made for caregiver sex, patient age, and patient income.

5. A review of the evidence supporting the added expense and effort entailed in special care units is R. Ohta and B. Ohta, "Special Care Units in Alzheimer's Disease Patients: A Critical Look," *Gerontologist* 28 (1988): 803–8.

6. Data from the National Nursing Home Survey (last completed in 1987) showed that 47 percent of those in nursing homes carry the diagnosis of dementia, and an additional 16 percent are characterized as disoriented or having decreased memory. (U.S. Senate Special Committee on Aging, *Aging America: Trends and Projections*. US DHHS: Washington, D.C., 1988.) One study found that as many as 94 percent of residents have mental disorders, principally dementia. P. Drinka and T. Howell, "The Burden of Mental Disorders in the Nursing Home," *Journal of the American Geriatrics Society* 39 (1991): 730–31.

7. Two influential, muckraking, journalistic accounts of nursing home life are Mary Mendelsohn, *Tender Loving Greed* (New York: Knopf, 1974) and Bruce Vladeck, *Unloving Care: The Nursing Home Tragedy* (New York: Basic Books, 1990). The Institute of Medicine's recommendations on nursing home care were published as *Improving the Quality of Care in Nursing Homes* (Washington, D.C.: National Academy Press, 1986).

8. For a description of nursing home life from the point of view of the residents, see Tracy Kidder, *Old Friends* (Boston: Houghton Mifflin, 1993).

9. The work on caregiving for the elderly in general and for demented individuals in particular indicates that approximately 80 percent of help in the community is provided by family members, principally daughters and wives. See E. Brody, "The Informal Support System and the Health of the Future Aged," in N. Wilson, ed., *Aging 2000: Our Health Care Destiny* (New York: Springer Verlag, 1985, pp. 174–89).

10. Many older Americans continue to believe that Medicare will pay for a nursing home if they need one. In fact, Medicare pays only about 2 percent of nursing home costs. Medicare pays for one hundred days of skilled nursing care (twenty days in full, eighty days with a copayment) for those select individuals who require skilled nursing care on a regular basis. Medicaid, on the other hand, pays in full for nursing home care for those individuals whose low income qualifies them for Medicaid. The net result is that Medicaid pays 42 percent of all expenditures on nursing home care. The remainder is paid for by a few other

government programs (principally the Veterans Administration, for eligible veterans), private long-term care insurance, and by the elderly themselves out of pocket. What this means is that affluent elderly start out paying for nursing home care privately, but even among the relatively well off, most cannot afford the $30,000 to $50,000 a year for a nursing home for very long. Once these individuals have run out of money, they become eligible for Medicaid, which takes over the payment of the nursing home. See Health and Public Policy Committee, American College of Physicians, "Financing Long-Term Care," *Annals of Internal Medicine* 108 (1988): 279–88.

11. An interesting ethnographic study of nursing home life, from the point of view of nursing assistants, is Timothy Diamond, *Making Gray Gold: Narratives of Nursing Home Care* (Chicago: University of Chicago Press, 1992).

12. Aggressive behavior—spitting, kicking, biting, verbal abuse—has been reported to occur in 21 to 43 percent of outpatients with dementia. See T. Howell and D. Watts, "Behavioral Complications of Dementia: A Clinical Approach for the General Internist," *Journal of General Internal Medicine* 5 (1990): 431–37.

13. A major study of the efficacy of CPR in the elderly in general and in the nursing home population in particular is D. Murphy, A. Murray, B. Robinson, and E. Campion, "Outcomes of Cardiopulmonary Resuscitation in the Elderly," *Annals of Internal Medicine* 111 (1989): 199–205. Dr. Murphy has argued, based on this and other studies, that the standard of care for residents of nursing homes should be *not* to attempt resuscitation, unless they or their families specifically demand otherwise. See Donald Murphy, "Do-Not-Resuscitate Orders: Time for Reappraisal in Long-Term Care Institutions," *Journal of the American Medical Association* 260 (1990): 2098–2101.

14. A good discussion of the legal aspects of withdrawing and withholding care is Robert Weir, "Decisions to Abate Life-Sustaining Treatment for Nonautonomous Patients," *Journal of the American Medical Association* 264 (1990): 1846–53.

15. Two well-known cases of competent patients refusing therapy are *Bouvia* v. *Superior Court*, in which a quadriplegic woman successfully sued to have her feeding tube removed, and *Bartling* v. *Superior Court*, in which an older man with lung cancer petitioned for the removal of a respirator, both cases from California. The correct description of these patients is "decision capable."

16. Several well-known cases of refusal of therapy for incompetent patients include *Brophy* v. *NE Sinai*, centering around removal of a feeding tube, and the Brother Fox case (*Eichner* v. *Dillon*), dealing with dialysis. The literature dealing with the rights of incompetent patients

is well summarized in R. Weir and L. Gostin, "Decisions to Abate Life-Sustaining Treatment for Nonautonomous Patients," *Journal of the American Medical Association* 264 (1990): 1846–53.

17. Nancy Beth Cruzan was in an automobile accident that left her in a persistent vegetative state. Her parents petitioned the courts in her home state of Missouri to discontinue her feeding tube. The Missouri court ruled that the parents could only authorize withdrawal of the feeding tube if they could produce "clear and convincing evidence" that their daughter would not have wanted artificial nutrition under the circumstances, which the court felt they had not supplied. The US Supreme Court upheld the Missouri court's decision. Subsequently, the Cruzans were able to find witnesses who stated that Nancy Beth had in fact stated something to the effect that she would not want to be maintained in a vegetative state, and the court then allowed the removal of the feeding tube.

■ **CHAPTER 8:** *Alzheimer's Disease in the Eyes of America*

1. The comments about TB (and those about cancer that follow) draw heavily from the insightful work of Susan Sontag, *Illness as Metaphor* (New York: Vintage, 1979). I elaborate on the role of metaphor in society, as Sontag's book does not fully explain the psychological purpose served by seeing TB as a disease of passion, so I am responsible for any weak links in the argument.

2. Again I am indebted to Susan Sontag. But once more I have begun with her observations about how cancer is viewed and interpreted them in light of what sociologists call representative characters, a public image that helps define the kinds of personality traits that it is desirable to develop.

3. Sontag, *Illness as Metaphor* (New York: Vintage, 1979), p. 57.

4. N. Mace and P. Rabins, *The 36-Hour Day* (Baltimore, Md.: Johns Hopkins University Press, rev. ed., 1991).

5. Jaber Gubrium, *Oldtimers and Alzheimer's: The Descriptive Organization of Senility* (Greenwich, Conn.: Jai Alai Press, 1986).

6. M. Vitez, "America's Aging Population Continues to Swell and Life Spans Climb," *Philadelphia Inquirer,* October 2, 1995.

7. Judy Foreman, "U.S. Elderly Outlive Their Peers Abroad," *Boston Globe,* June 20, 1995, p. 4.

8. N. Walfoort, "A New Age for Old Age: Needs of Elderly Will Shape Future," *Louisville, Ky., Courier-Journal,* January 8, 1995, p. 1A.

9. N. Walfoort, "A New Age for Old Age: Many May Want or Need to Work Beyond Age 65," *Louisville, Ky., Courier-Journal,* January 9, 1995, p. 1B.

10. Gail Wilensky, "The Score on Medicare Reform—Minus the Hype and Hyperbole," *New England Journal of Medicine* 333 (1995): 1774–77.

11. My conclusions about the view of aging and of dementia in the news media derives from a review of all 217 articles appearing in the CD-Rom News media collection, using the key words "elderly persons," "aging," and "Alzheimer's disease" for the period December 1994 through November 1995.

12. See Luigi Carnaro, *The Art of Living* (Milwaukee: William Butler, 1918).

13. See J. Fries, G. Singh, D. Morfeld, et al., "Running and the Development of Disability with Age," *Annals of Internal Medicine* 121 (1994): 502–9, and also R. Donahue, R. Abbott, D. Reed, and K. Yano, "Physical Activity and Coronary Heart Disease in Middle-Aged and Elderly Men; the Honolulu Heart Program," *American Journal of Public Health* 78 (1988): 683–85.

14. M. Fiatarone, E. Marks, N. Ryan, et al., "High-Intensity Strength Training in Nonagenarians: Effects on Skeletal Muscle," *Journal of the American Medical Association* 263 (1990): 329–34.

15. John Morley, "Nutrition in the Elderly," *Annals of Internal Medicine* 109 (1988): 890–904.

16. Debra Gordon, "Good Nutrition Can Make Dramatic Difference in Quality of Life for Seniors," *The Virginian-Pilot*, April 7, 1995.

17. "Aging Gracefully," *St. Louis Post-Dispatch,* July 13, 1995, p. 1A.

18. Elsa Arnett, "Single Physical Test Predicts Which People Will Become Disabled," Knight-Ridder Washington Bureau, March 1, 1995. The actual study is J. Guralnik, L. Ferrucci, E. Simonsick, et al., "Lower-Extremity Function in Persons Over the Age of 70 Years as a Predictor of Subsequent Disability," *New England Journal of Medicine* 332 (1995): 556–61.

19. Thierry Cagnol, "Chocolate, Champagne for World's Oldest Person, 120," Reuters, February 2, 1995.

20. John Schieszer, "Happy Birthday into Your 100s? Science Is Studying How," *St. Louis Post-Dispatch,* April 16, 1996, p. 16.

21. Rachel Jones, "Elderly Urged to Stay Healthy Longer by Exercising Preventive Care," Knight-Ridder Washington Bureau, May 2, 1995.

22. Theresa Tighe, "Assisted Living Opens Doors for the Elderly," *St. Louis Post-Dispatch,* March 26, 1995, p. 1D.

23. Jerome Avorn and Evelyn Langer, "Induced Disability in Nursing Home Patients: A Controlled Trial," *Journal of the American Geriatrics Society* 30 (1982): 397–400.

24. Hugh McCann, "Nuns' Austere Habits Make Them a Blessing to Brain Research," *Detroit News,* June 19, 1995, p. E1.

25. D. Snowdon, S. Kemper, J. Mortimer, et al., "Linguistic Ability in Early Life and Cognitive Function and Alzheimer's Disease in Late Life: Findings from the Nun Study," *Journal of the American Medical Association* 275 (1996): 528–32.

26. Y. Stern, B. Gurland, T. Tatemichi, et al., "Influence of Education and Occupation on the Incidence of Alzheimer's Disease," *Journal of the American Medical Association* 271 (1994): 1004–10.

27. Doug Adams, "Older Workers Face New Challenges: The Search Is More Difficult and Stressful for Older Job Seekers," *Indianapolis Star,* May 3, 1995, p. D1.

28. A study of forty-seven individuals over time was reported by James Birren, ed., in *Human Aging I: A Biological and Behavioral Study* (Rockville, Md: National Institute of Mental Health, 1971). This study found that only those individuals with significant physical problems developed cognitive deficits. A larger longitudinal study, E. Busse and G. Maddox, *The Duke Longitudinal Studies of Normal Aging, 1955–1980* (New York: Springer, 1985), demonstrated that mental function was preserved in the majority of older subjects, *until the eighth decade.*

29. V. Hachinski, "Preventable Senility: A Call for Action Against the Vascular Dementias," *Lancet* 340 (1992): 645–8.

30. Gordon Slovut, "Blood Test May Predict Likelihood of Alzheimer's, Report Says," *Star Tribune: Newspaper of the Twin Cities,* April 26, 1995.

31. The medical article referred to is G. Small, J. Mazziotta, M. Collins, et al., "Apoprotein E Type 4 Allele and Critical Glucose Metabolism in Relatives at Risk for Familial Alzheimer's Disease," *Journal of the American Medical Association* 273 (1995): 942–47. The study actually looked at people with mild cognitive impairment *and* a first-degree relative with Alzheimer's disease, and found that those people with the apoE-ε4 allele were more likely to have asymmetry between the metabolism in the left and right parietal lobes of the brain (shown in another study to be associated with Alzheimer's disease) than those people without the apoE-ε4 allele.

32. David Gorham, "Brain Graft Help for Alzheimer's Shows Promise," *San Diego Union-Tribune,* June 8, 1995, pp. B1, 7, 8.

33. David Balingrud, "Major Piece of Alzheimer's Puzzle Found," *St. Petersburg Times,* June 29, 1995, p. 1A.

34. Richard Saltus, "Gene That Causes Early Alzheimer's Is Reported Found," *Boston Globe,* June 29, 1995.

35. Quoted in Patrick Howington, "Research Offers Hope in War on

Alzheimer's: Cure Still Elusive, but Scientists Claim Better Understanding," *Louisville, Ky., Courier-Journal,* December 27, 1994, p. 1A.

36. The series, appearing in *Long Island, N.Y., Newsday* and written by Laura Muha, was composed of four installments: "Care Givers' Tug-of-War" (April 16, 1995 p. A7), "One Day at a Time" (April 17, 1995, p. B3), "Four Sides of Caregiving" (April 18, 1995, p. B4), and "The Essence of Caregiving" (April 22, 1995, p. B1).

37. Michael Norman, "Living Too Long," *New York Times Magazine,* January 14, 1996, pp. 36–38.

38. Laura Blumenfeld, "Time Took Her Family Away, and Alzheimer's Has Given Them Back to Her: A Story About the Mind and Eternity," *Washington Post,* October 15, 1995, p. F1.

39. Daniel Berger, "Murder-Suicide Cases Could Be on Increase," *Tampa Tribune,* February 22, 1995, p. 7.

40. Lynda Hurst, "Nightmare of Dementia: 40,000 Living in Homes for Elderly Suffer from Mental Illness," *Toronto Star,* March 18, 1995, p. A1.

41. This is discussed in detail in the chapter "Family Caregiving and the Ethics of Behavior Control," in Stephen Post, *The Moral Challenge of Alzheimer Disease* (Baltimore, Md.: Johns Hopkins University Press, 1995), pp. 42–61. Post comments that "the family is often uniquely solicitous because of a deeply personal memory of and gratitude toward the affected person before the onset of illness." He also cites evidence that caregiver spouses continue to value their mate as a "unique person" despite impairment. Finally, he notes that some individuals in our society, particularly women, "may find caregiving roles to be profoundly meaningful and even inspiring."

42. Janet Rae-Dupree, "Mice Genetically Altered to Develop Alzheimer's Suffer the Same Memory Loss as Humans," *San Jose Mercury News,* June 6, 1995.

43. The study, conducted by the UCLA Gerontology Institute in 1993, found that 64 percent of the 6,800 people polled believed TV does not do a good job of portraying old people. Seventy-eight percent felt there should be more programs featuring older people. Moreover, adults fifty-five and over watch more television than any other age group. What was far from clear was whether the fifty-five plus group wanted to see programs with older characters. Reported by K. Littlefield, "Gray Power," *The Orange County Register,* March 5, 1995, p. F8.

44. Mike Featherstone and Mike Hepworth, "Images of Positive Aging: A Case Study of *Retirement Choice Magazine,*" in Mike Featherstone and Andrew Wernick, eds., *Images of Aging: Cultural Representations of Later Life* (London: Routledge, 1995). A whole host of magazines have sprung up targeted to the older reader (typically defined as over fifty,

but sometimes intended for those over sixty-five). The only one I have encountered that consistently addresses the more sober side of aging is *Answers: The Magazine for Adult Children of Aging Parents.* A sample issue (Summer 1996) included columns on checking up on frail parents, Alzheimer's disease, and strategies for paying nursing home costs. The feature articles were on falling and on a battle for conservatorship of a parent with dementia.

45. George Maddox, director of the Long Term Care Resources Program at Duke University, contrasted the "new view" of age as a period of continued growth with the "old approach" in which aging was regarded as "a process of decline leading to death." See Jeff Kunerth, "Researcher: Aging Has New Meaning," *Orlando Sentinel,* April 5, 1995, p. D1.

46. Betty Friedan, *The Fountain of Age* (New York: Simon & Schuster, 1993).

47. Ken Dychtwald and Joe Flower, *Age Wave: The Challenges and Opportunities of an Aging America* (Los Angeles: Jeremy P. Tarcher, 1989).

48. Gail Sheehy, *New Passages: Mapping Your Life Across Time* (New York: Random House, 1995).

49. Thomas Cole, *The Journey of Life: A Cultural History of Aging in America* (New York: Cambridge University Press, 1992). The first and most eminent of the debunkers was Robert Butler, whose book *Why Survive?* (New York: Harper and Row, 1975) won the Pulitzer Prize.

50. Daniel Callahan discusses this at length in his seminal book, *Setting Limits. Medical Goals in an Aging Society* (New York: Simon & Schuster, 1987). He concludes that "both the old and the young turn out to need the same thing: a way of imaginatively and reflectively integrating their individual life stages into the larger cycle of the generations." He believes that the old can find meaning only in "service to the young." It is again unclear that "the unique capacity of the elderly to see the way past, present, and future interact" is applicable to the demented.

51. See Thomas Cole, "The 'Enlightened' View of Aging: Victorian Morality in a New Key," in T. Cole and S. Gadow, eds., *What Does It Mean to Grow Old?* (Durham, N.C.: Duke University Press, 1986), pp. 117–30.

52. See Thomas Cole, "The 'Enlightened' View of Aging: Victorian Morality in a New Key," in T. Cole and S. Gadow, eds. *What Does It Mean to Grow Old?* (Durham, N.C.: Duke University Press, 1986), p. 123.

53. R. Bellah, R. Madsen, et al., *Habits of the Heart: Individualism and Commitment in American Life* (New York: Harper and Row, 1986).

54. The collapse of the liberal consensus is the theme of Godfrey

Hodgson's book, *America in Our Time: From World War II to Nixon. What Happened and Why* (New York: Doubleday, 1976).

55. A nice discussion of what, in the bioethics jargon, has been called *executional autonomy* versus *decisional autonomy* is by L. McCullough, N. Wilson, J. Rhymes, and T. Teasdale, "Managing the Conceptual and Ethical Dimensions of Long-Term Care Decision-Making: A Preventive Ethics Approach," in L. McCullough and N. Wilson, eds., *Long-Term Care Decisions: Ethical and Conceptual Dimensions* (Baltimore, Md.: Johns Hopkins University Press 1995), pp. 221–40.

■ CHAPTER 9: *Midnight*

1. Living wills have been around since 1969. They were promulgated by the Society for the Right to Die, renamed Choice in Dying. A book about living wills and other forms of advance planning is T. Hill and D. Shirley, *A Good Death: Taking More Control at the End of Your Life* (New York: Addison-Wesley, 1992).

2. See, for example, L. Emanuel and E. Emanuel, "The Medical Directive: A New Comprehensive Advance Care Document," *Journal of the American Medical Association* 261 (1989): 3288–93 as well as their more recent article, L. Emanuel, M. Barry, J. Stoeckle, et al., "Advance Directives for Medical Care—a Case for Greater Use," *New England Journal of Medicine* 324 (1991): 889–95. For a discussion of the weaknesses of this type of advance directive, see Allan Brett, "Limitation of Listing Specific Medical Interventions in Advance Directives," *Journal of the American Medical Association* 266 (1991): 825–28.

3. It is important to distinguish here between the effect of age alone and the effect of chronic illness. In study after study, age alone is of little importance in determining the efficacy of treatment. For example, thrombolytic agents, or clot busters, were initially given to heart attack patients only if they were younger than sixty-five or seventy. Careful studies disclosed that, if anything, older people derived even more benefit from these drugs than younger people, probably because their heart attacks tended to be more severe and the Roto-Rooter effect was correspondingly more dramatic. But functional status—the patient's ability to care for himself, which is inversely associated with the number of chronic diseases he has—is strongly correlated with the outcome of a variety of treatments such as intensive care. See, for example, S. Mayer-Oakes, R. Oye, B. Leak, et al., "Predictors of Mortality in older Patients Following Medical Intensive Care: The Importance of Functional Status," *Journal of the American Geriatrics Society* 39 (1991): 862–68.

4. A study of lucid dying patients who were unable to eat or drink found that thirst and hunger were rare. Any thirst or hunger that did exist was readily alleviated with ice chips or an occasional sip of juice. See

R. McCann, W. Hall, and A. Groth-Juncker, "Comfort Care for Terminally Ill Patients: the Appropriate Use of Nutrition and Hydration," *Journal of the American Medical Association* 272 (1994): 1263–66. An article making the argument that *artificial* nutrition and hydration have little in common with eating and drinking is J. Slomka, "What Do Apple Pie and Motherhood Have to Do with Feeding Tubes and Caring for the Patient?" *Archives of Internal Medicine* 155 (1995): 1258–63.

5. Withholding of "food and fluids," an unfortunate shorthand for withholding artificial nutrition and hydration from a patient who cannot eat or drink, has been a highly controversial area for the last several years. Two landmark cases are *Brophy* and *Cruzan*. In *Brophy*, the Massachusetts Supreme Judicial Court authorized the removal of a feeding tube from Paul Brophy, a firefighter in a persistent vegetative state after a blood vessel ruptured in his brain, in accordance with the request of his observant Catholic wife. In *Cruzan*, the U.S. Supreme Court upheld the ruling of a Missouri state court, which, in turn, had declared constitutional Missouri legislation that insisted treatment could be withheld from incompetent patients only if there was "clear and convincing" evidence that the patient would have wanted the treatment withheld. The Supreme Court did not require a clear and convincing evidence standard; it simply supported the right of individual state legislatures to set their own standards. To date, only Missouri and New York have such stringent standards. It is worth mentioning that after the Supreme Court ruling, the Cruzan family managed to produce a witness who satisfied the Missouri court that Nancy Cruzan, before she lapsed into a vegetative state as a result of a car accident when she was twenty-one, had stated she would not wish to be maintained in such a condition. Nancy's feeding tube was withdrawn, and she died.

6. The phenomenon of adverse consequences of hospitalization in the elderly is well described. Efforts to prevent functional decline have met with limited success: only one study has reported that patients treated on a special unit could hope to be discharged at a level near their prehospitalization state. (C. Landefeld, R. Palmer, D. Kresevic, et al., "A Randomized Trial of Care in a Hospital Medical Unit Especially Designed to Improve the Functional Outcomes of Acutely Ill Older Patients," *New England Journal of Medicine* 332 [1995]: 1238–44.) See also articles by M. Gillick, N. Serrell, and L. Gillick, "Adverse Consequences of Hospitalization in the Elderly," *Social Science and Medicine* 16 (1982): 1033–38 and by M. Creditor, "Hazards of Hospitalization in the Elderly," *Annals of Internal Medicine* 118 (1993): 219–23.

7. See L. Volicer, Y. Rheaume, J. Brown, et al., "Hospice Approach to the Treatment of Patients with Advanced Dementia of the Alzheimer Type," *Journal of the American Medical Association* 256 (1986): 2210–13.

8. Deuteronomy 22:5. This translation is from Jeffrey Tigay, ed., *The JPS Torah Commentary* (Philadelphia: Jewish Publication Society, 1996).

9. S. Mitchell, D. Kiely, and L. Lipsitz, "The Risk Factors and Impact on Survival of Feeding Tube Placement in Nursing Home Residents with Severe Cognitive Impairment," *Archives of Internal Medicine* 157 (1997), 327–32.

10. A recent portrait of the various forms death may take is to be found in Sherwin Nuland's *How We Die* (New York: Knopf, 1994).

■ *Epilogue*

1. See R. Henig, *The Myth of Senility*, rev. ed., (New York: AARP Books, 1986).

2. Allen Buchanan and Dan Brock, "Advance Directives, Personhood, and Personal Identity," in A. Buchanan and D. Brock, *Deciding for Others: The Ethics of Surrogate Decision-Making* (Cambridge: Cambridge University Press, 1989), argue that personal identity is maintained provided that there is evidence of *psychological continuity*. From this point of view, the individual with advanced dementia who has "such extensive, permanent neurological damage that the patient's memory has been destroyed, his or her cognitive processes have been virtually obliterated, and all that remains is basic perceptual awareness" has lost all personhood. "He may still be capable of feeling pain and physical pleasure, although of fleeting and rudimentary sorts." Buchanan and Brock argue that the living being who remains is not a person at all, and hence not a *different* person.

3. Even Eric Cassell, in his seminal work *The Nature of Suffering and the Goals of Medicine* (New York: Oxford University Press, 1991), concludes that the major goal of medicine is the relief of suffering. He agrees with me about the distinction between acute and chronic illness, and speaks of "illness" when he means the patient's experience of the objective "disease," but is perhaps more sanguine than I am about the extent to which physicians are able to relieve all suffering. He makes the important point, however, that alleviation from suffering is achieved at least as often by talking to patients, establishing a relationship with them, and helping them cope as it is by prescribing medications.

4. Tuberculosis is having somewhat of a resurgence with the AIDS epidemic. TB bacteria resistant to all existing antibiotics have made their appearance—see Frank Ryan, *The Forgotten Plague* (Boston: Little, Brown, 1994). But my point is that yesterday's chronic illnesses can sometimes metamorphose into today's acute illnesses.

Index